USMLE STEP 2 CK

Neurology & Psychiatry

In Your Pocket

✓ Study guide for the USMLE STEP 2 CK exam.

✓ Prepare for your shelf examination.

✓ Be ready for your inpatient rotation.

Gregory J. Fernandez M.D.

First Edition, 2016
Author & Editor: Gregory J. Fernandez, M.D.
Publisher: M.D. Educational Services
Peer-reviewers:　Neurology, Dr. Mohd Ishtiayaq Khan;
　　　　　　　　Psychiatry, Dr. Hasnain Afzal
Book Design: Marie Meyer
Copyediting: Editage Cactus Communications

DISCLAIMER: The author, editor, publisher, and staff members have taken care to confirm the accuracy of the information present in this publication. The context of the books entirety, is believed to be reliable in accordance with the standards accepted at the time of publication. However, readers are encouraged to confirm the information and conduct their own research for clarification of all the information present within this book. No one involved in creating this book is responsible for errors or omissions or for any consequences from application of the information in this book. There is no warranty, expressed or implied, with respect to the completeness or accuracy of the contents of this publication. Neither the editor, nor the author assumes any liability for any injury and/or damage to persons or property arising from the content of this publication. Application of this information in a particular situation remains the professional responsibility of the practitioner; the clinical treatments or information described and recommended may not be considered absolute and universal recommendations. It is the responsibility of the health care provider to ascertain the FDA status of each drug used or device planned for use in their clinical practice. The purpose of this books, is to be used as a study guide for medical examinations. Please consult with attending physicians for any medical decisions.

ISBN-13: 978-1540471802

ISBN-10: 1540471802

This book is gratefully dedicated to my wife. Thank you for your support and always being there for me. Thank you for your kindness, your devotion, and your endless selflessness support. I love you… Thank you mother, father, step-mother, brothers, friends, and family for all your encouragement and endless love. Best of luck to all the medical dreamers, the road is long and I hope my book helps you through this journey. All the best…

How to Use
"Neurology & Psychiatry In Your Pocket"

Neurology & Psychiatry In Your Pocket is a study guide for the USMLE STEP 2 CK exam that you can also use to prepare for your shelf examination and to get ready for your inpatient rotation. It is part of a series, each dealing with a different subject or sub-specialty, focusing on vital clinical knowledge.

The subjects and topics within neurology and psychiatry are called out in large, colored type. These items are also included in the Table of Contents for ease of access.

Many subjects also contain sub-subjects that are also called out in bold, blue type either as bulleted items or in-line with the text, as appropriate. They are all referenced in the index.

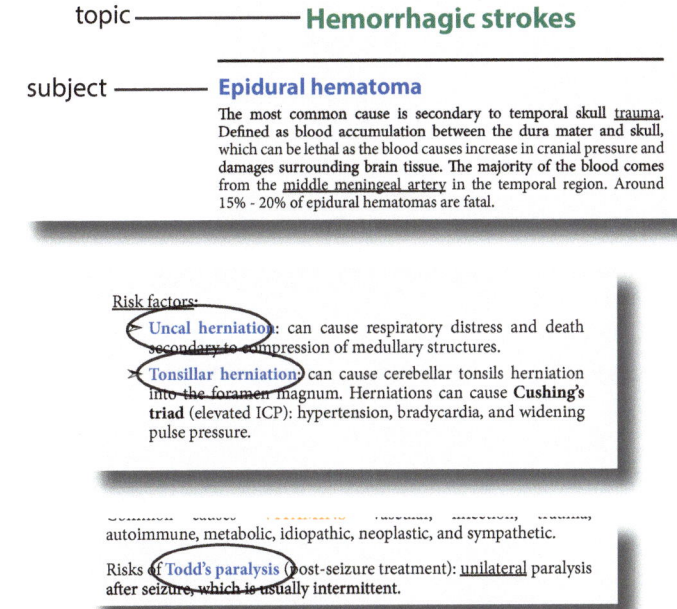

topic ——————— **Hemorrhagic strokes**

subject ——————— **Epidural hematoma**
The most common cause is secondary to temporal skull <u>trauma</u>. Defined as blood accumulation between the dura mater and skull, which can be lethal as the blood causes increase in cranial pressure and damages surrounding brain tissue. The majority of the blood comes from the <u>middle meningeal artery</u> in the temporal region. Around 15% - 20% of epidural hematomas are fatal.

Risk factors:
> **Uncal herniation**: can cause respiratory distress and death secondary to compression of medullary structures.
> **Tonsillar herniation** can cause cerebellar tonsils herniation into the foramen magnum. Herniations can cause **Cushing's triad** (elevated ICP): hypertension, bradycardia, and widening pulse pressure.

Common causes ...., ..., ..., autoimmune, metabolic, idiopathic, neoplastic, and sympathetic.

Risks of **Todd's paralysis** (post-seizure treatment): <u>unilateral</u> paralysis after seizure, which is usually intermittent.

Presentation of clinical history and physical exam (Hx/PE), step-by-step diagnosis, and treatment plan are indicated by bold red headings.

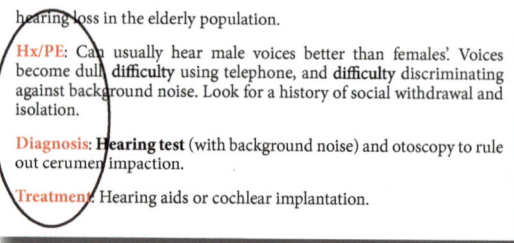

hearing loss in the elderly population.

Hx/PE: Can usually hear male voices better than females'. Voices become dull, **difficulty** using telephone, and **difficulty** discriminating against background noise. Look for a history of social withdrawal and isolation.

Diagnosis: **Hearing test** (with background noise) and otoscopy to rule out cerumen impaction.

Treatment: Hearing aids or cochlear implantation.

Procedures, triads, pathology, medications, antibodies and findings are called out in bold text. These items are also included in the index.

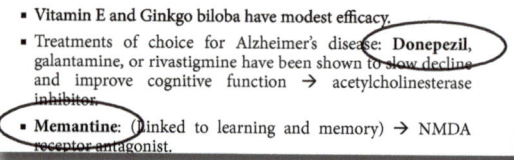

- Vitamin E and Ginkgo biloba have modest efficacy.
- Treatments of choice for Alzheimer's disease: **Donepezil**, galantamine, or rivastigmine have been shown to slow decline and improve cognitive function → acetylcholinesterase inhibitor.
- **Memantine**: (linked to learning and memory) → NMDA receptor antagonist.

Reflexes, signs and maneuvers are shown in purple text.

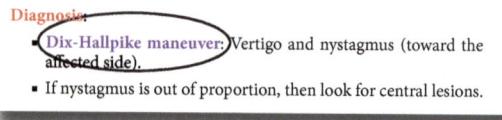

Diagnosis:
- Dix-Hallpike maneuver: Vertigo and nystagmus (toward the affected side).
- If nystagmus is out of proportion, then look for central lesions.

Mnemonics and key words are shown in orange text.

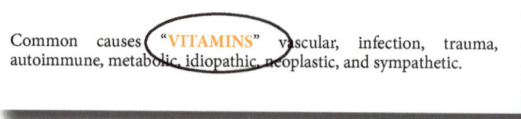

Common causes "VITAMINS" vascular, infection, trauma, autoimmune, metabolic, idiopathic, neoplastic, and sympathetic.

And, finally, for the avoidance of doubt, circumstances that amount to a medical emergency are flagged with warning.

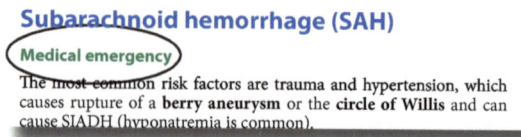

Subarachnoid hemorrhage (SAH)

Medical emergency

The most common risk factors are trauma and hypertension, which causes rupture of a **berry aneurysm** or the **circle of Willis** and can cause SIADH (hyponatremia is common).

Neurology
Table of Contents

Psychiatry
Table of Contents

Neurology

Hemorrhagic strokes

Epidural hematoma

The most common cause is secondary to temporal skull trauma. Defined as blood accumulation between the dura mater and skull, which can be lethal as the blood causes increase in cranial pressure and damages surrounding brain tissue. The majority of the blood comes from the middle meningeal artery in the temporal region. Around 15% - 20% of epidural hematomas are fatal.

Hx/PE: Typical patterns are altered mental status (AMS), headache (moderate to severe), tachycardia, tachypnea, and loss of consciousness followed by "lucid intervals."

Risk factors:

➤ Uncal herniation: can cause respiratory distress and death secondary to compression of medullary structures.

➤ Tonsillar herniation: can cause cerebellar tonsils herniation into the foramen magnum. Herniations can cause **Cushing's triad** (elevated ICP): hypertension, bradycardia, and widening pulse pressure.

Diagnosis:

■ First step is stabilization of patient. Focus on assessing patient's airway, breathing, blood pressure control, and increased intracranial pressure.

- First study: head CT scan without contrast ("**lens-shaped**" or convex hyperdensity that does <u>not</u> cross suture lines).
  - Head CT scan distinguishes between hemorrhagic and ischemic strokes.
- Basic orders:
  - CBC: monitor infection, hematocrit, and platelets.
  - PT/INR, PTT, and bleeding time: identify any bleeding disorders.
  - Electrolytes, glucose, and BUN/Cr ratio: monitor metabolic processes that may complicate the clinical course.

Treatment:
- If signs or symptoms of increased intracranial pressure (ICP), this is a **medical emergency**.
  - Focused on assessing patient's airway, breathing capability, and blood pressure control.
- <u>Small hematoma</u> (with no elevated ICP) can be treated without surgery and clinically monitored for worsening signs and symptoms.
- <u>Larger hematoma</u> or solid blood clots (>1 cm) may require surgery (**burr hole** or **craniotomy**).
- A combination of techniques and medications can be used to decrease ICP; including elevating head of bed to 30 degrees, hyperventilation (fastest response in lowering ICP), and IV mannitol (take effect in 15-30 minutes). Hyperventilation is more realistic if the patient is intubated.
- <u>Cushing triad</u> (if develops), will need intubation (hyperventilate), IV mannitol, and blood pressure control.
- Consult neurology and place the patient under aspiration precautions.

<u>Prophylaxis</u>: for seizures (phenytoin [controversial]), vasospasms (nimodipine), elevated blood pressure (IV β-blockers, if no contraindications), and stress ulcers (PPIs).

Note:
- ✓Control hypertension with IV β-blockers (systolic blood

pressure target range 140-160 mmHg; not lower to help maintain cerebral perfusion pressure).

✓Need a complete assessment after head trauma, including a complete neurological examination.

Subdural hematoma

This is also known as shaken baby syndrome in children. Slower progression of symptoms compared to epidural hematoma and found in elderly patients with head trauma, "shaken babies", and alcoholics. Involves the <u>bridging veins</u>, and the hematoma can be seen between the dura mater and arachnoid membrane.

Hx/PE: Associated symptoms are headaches, AMS, confusion, seizures, and loss of consciousness.

Diagnosis:

- First step is stabilization of patient.
- First study: head CT scan without contrast ("crescent-shape" or concave hyperdensity and <u>can</u> cross suture lines).
- Order basic labs: CBC, electrolytes, glucose, PT/INR, PTT, bleeding time, and BUN/Cr ratio.
- If suspected child abuse, the first steps are stabilization, treatment, hospitalization, and then contact child protective services.

Treatment:

- May or may not require surgery, which will depend on the size of hematoma and overall clinical picture.
- If large hematoma (>1 cm), consider burr hole or craniotomy.
- Elevated ICP: consider steroids (controversial), head elevation, hyperventilation, and mannitol.

Prophylaxis: for seizures (phenytoin [controversial]), vasospasms (nimodipine), elevated blood pressure (IV β blockers), and stress ulcers (PPIs).

Note:

✓Burr hole or craniotomy always carry risks of mortality, infection, and hemorrhage.

✓Keep in mind that generally, loss of consciousness usually requires work-up with head CT scan without contrast.

Subarachnoid hemorrhage (SAH)

Medical emergency

The most common risk factors are trauma and hypertension, which causes rupture of a **berry aneurysm** or the **circle of Willis** and can cause SIADH (hyponatremia is common).

Hx/PE: Sudden onset of headache ("worst headache of my life"), thunderclap headache, neck stiffness, and photophobia.

Note: Photophobia and neck stiffness is common in meningitis (gradual onset) and SAH (sudden onset).

Diagnosis:

- If unstable, first steps are to control blood pressure, airway, and intracranial pressure.
- Then, order head CT scan without contrast (most sensitive if done <12 hours of onset).
- If head CT scan is negative, with high suspicion or >12 hours since onset of hemorrhage, then perform lumbar puncture (more sensitive if >12 hours).
  - Lumbar puncture: RBCs/yellow/**xanthochromia**/ increased proteins/increased ICP.
  - Traumatic lumbar puncture can also cause elevated RBCs, however, the supernatant is clear after centrifugation in traumatic lumbar puncture; unlike after a real hemorrhage which stays yellow.
- Order basic labs: CBC, electrolytes, glucose, PT/INR, PTT, bleeding time, and BUN/Cr ratio.
- Once SAH is diagnosed, perform CT angiography with 3D reconstruction.
- Call neurosurgery (STAT), if either high suspicion or positive radiological findings.

Note: xanthochromia only lasts about 24–36 hours (reabsorbed).

Treatment:

- Control hypertension with IV β-blockers (systolic blood pressure target range 140–160 but not lower to help maintain cerebral perfusion pressure).
- Decrease ICP with head elevation, hyperventilation (fast), mannitol (15-30 minutes), and/or burr hole.
- Prevent vasospasm with nimodipine (calcium blocker).
- Prevent seizures with phenytoin (controversial).
- Prevent stress ulcers with PPIs.
- If patient is on warfarin (review all medications) and will need FFP infusion.
- **Surgical clipping** (definitive treatment).

Note: Sublingual anti-hypertensive medications are not recommended, as these medications might lower blood pressure too rapidly (can cause brain hypoperfusion), and difficult to control the target blood pressure. IV medications are used for control that is more precise.

Ischemic strokes

Ischemic stroke

Accounts for 80% of all strokes and caused by vascular blockage to the blood supply to brain. The highest single risk factor is hypertension. They are rare in women under 50 years of age (secondary to estrogen protection). Patients will need an extensive work-up to rule out secondary causes.

Risk factors: hypertension (highest risk factor), advanced age, smoking, diabetes, males, hypercoagulability, atrial fibrillation, hyperlipidemia, obesity, and previous TIA.

Stroke locations and symptoms:

- ➤ **Middle cerebral artery (MCA):** associated with aphasia, sensory and motor loss of the arms and face, and involvement of the Broca's (brodmann area 44 and 45) and Wernicke's areas (brodmann area 22). The left MCA is the dominant side and commonly presents with aphasia.

➤ **Anterior cerebral artery (ACA)**: associated with personality changes, sensory and motor loss to the lower extremities, and urinary and fecal incontinence.

➤ **Posterior cerebral artery (PCA):** associated with visual changes, occipital cortex, and cranial nerve III.

➤ **Basilar artery stroke:** this stroke type is associated with poor prognosis and involves a posterior stroke affecting the pons and the cerebellum. "**Locked-in-syndrome**" can be caused by damage to the pons. Patients are aware but cannot communicate verbally or conduct muscle movements, except for eye movements.

➤ **Lacunar stroke:** usually creates a pure motor (most common type of lucunar stroke, about 35%-50%) or a pure sensory dysfunction (numbness, abnormal sensation, or perception of pain). There are other types of lacunar strokes. Usually affects the posterior limb of the internal capsule or the thalamus. Can have silent lacunar stroke where there are no symptoms.

Note:

✓ The anterior circulation comprises the MCA and ACA.

✓ The posterior circulation is innervated by the basilar artery and PCA.

Diagnosis:

- First step is always stabilization of patient.

- First test: obtain a head CT scan w/o contrast (lesion appears black). Acute ischemic strokes might not be visible on head CT scan and will need to order head MRI/MRA (most sensitive for ischemic stroke). Time is very important here and this should be done even before a mini-mental status examination (MMSE).

- Order basic labs: carotid Doppler, PTT, PT/INR, platelets, bleeding time, glucose level, EKG, echocardiogram, and lipid panel to help rule out other pathologies.

- Neurological tests while hospitalized should be done every hour during the first 24 hours.

- Initially place NPO and later will need a swallow study to determine if they can tolerate PO intake.
- Place aspiration precautions and in a semi-upright position.
- PPIs help with stress ulcers.

Treatment:

- tPA should be the first medication given and can be administered within the first 3 hours, after ruling out contraindications:

  Blood pressure >185/110 (stage 3), <18 years of age, glucose <40 or >400, platelets <100,000, if _ever_ had cranial hemorrhage, surgery within 2 weeks, stroke/head trauma within 3 months, INR >1.6, recent MI, seizures present at onset, and GI or urinary bleed within 3 weeks.

- Aspirin (ASA): decreases mortality if given within the first 48 hours and should be one of the first medications given.
- Clopidogrel can be added, if recurrent stroke occurs while on aspirin.
- Blood pressure cannot be higher than 185/105 (If higher, give IV β-blockers).
- Allow mild hypoxia and mild hypertension to maintain cerebral perfusion.
- Hypoglycemia and hyperglycemia need to be treated early in the evaluation.
  - Hyperglycemia in this case considered >200 mg/dL (give insulin).
- Fever greater than 100.4 F, should be treated with acetaminophen.
- Oxygen supplementation, if SaO2 <94%,
- Place patient NPO, as high risk of aspiration.
- IV normal saline infusion at 50 mL/hour, unless otherwise indicated.

Note: keep in mind that tPA can cause hemorrhagic strokes. If suspected, order a head CT scan w/o contrast.

Prevention considerations during hospitalization: DVT (SCDs), aspiration precautions, ambulation restrictions, swallow study, and frequent neurological status checks.

Long-term treatment:

- ASA <u>or</u> clopidogrel can be given even in the settings where tPA are contraindicated.
- Carotid endarterectomy if stenosis >70% and symptomatic.
  - Also, consider carotid angioplasty vs stenting.
- Add warfarin in cases of atrial fibrillation or hypercoagulable states.
  - INR goal range: 2–3 (normal) or 3–4 (patients with prosthetic valves).
- Management of diet, exercise, hypertension, diabetes, and dyslipidemia (statins).

Pathways

➤ **UMN lesions:** presents with spastic, increased DTR, increased muscle tone, and positive **Babinski sign**.

➤ **LMN lesions:** presents with flaccidity, decreased DTRs, and muscular atrophy.

➤ **Dorsal column medial lemniscus:** dorsal column → *medial lemniscus* (decussation) → primary motor cortex.

➤ **Spinothalamic:** pain and temperature pathway; with a *white commissure* (decussation) → Pain fibers: A-fibers (fast) and C-fibers (slow).

➤ **Lateral corticospinal tract:** motor pathway. UMN/LMN → *pyramidal* (decussation) → primary motor cortex.

➤ **Upper motor neuron lesion (facial):** motor cortex lesions affect the <u>contralateral</u> lower face.

➤ **Lower motor neuron lesion (facial):** <u>ipsilateral</u> upper and lower face.

Bell's palsy

Affects the *facial nucleus* resulting in dysfunction of the peripheral facial nerve (CN VII), leading to ipsilateral <u>upper</u> and <u>lower</u> facial paralysis. Also, loss of taste from the anterior two-thirds of the tongue (CN VII). Difficulty closing affected eye. Recovery takes about 1-6 months.

Risk factors: AIDS, diabetes, Lyme disease, EBV, and sarcoidosis.

Diagnosis:
- Clinical diagnosis: a helpful way to distinguish between a stroke and Bell's palsy is that patients with Bell's palsy cannot close their eye (on effected side) and absence of forehead furrow (cannot lift eyebrow). This can save patients from unnecessary thrombolytic treatment.
- In Lyme-endemic areas, will need further work-up to rule out Lyme disease.

Treatment:
- Treatment of choice: steroids (within 3 days of onset) and eye care (artificial tears) are the most important intervention.
- Antiviral medication (acyclovir). Antiviral medications are controversial.

Headaches

Types:
- Acute: seconds to minutes.
- Subacute: hours to days.
- Chronic: weeks to months.

Worrisome symptoms are severe headaches, acute or new onset, fever, onset after 40 years of age, changes in headache, posterior headache, and focal findings.

Migraines

The exact mechanism is unknown, but migraines are believed to be a neurovascular disorder or associated to hormonal changes, such as elevation of serotonin levels. Other factors can include genetic and environmental factors. They usually last longer than 2 hours but tend to be less than 48 hours.

<u>Triggers</u>: can be associated with consumption of red wine, cheese, chocolates, fasting, stress, menses, OCPs, bright light, and disrupted sleep patterns.

<u>Types</u>:
➤ **Classic migraines** (unilateral with aura).

➤ **Common migraines** (bilateral without aura).

Hx/PE: Symptoms can include unilateral or bilateral throbbing headache, photophobia, audiophobia, nausea, and vomiting.

Diagnosis:

- Clinical diagnosis.
- Patients should keep a diary documenting the headaches (frequency, duration, intensity, and associated symptoms).
- Rule out other pathologies, with the consideration of the following symptoms:
  - Jaw pain and visual loss: giant cell.
  - Photophobia: migraine, meningitis, or SAH.
  - Fever or rash: meningitis or encephalitis.
  - Stiff neck: SAH or meningitis.
  - Ocular pressure: glaucoma.
  - Weight loss: cerebral neoplasms or metastasis.
  - Papillary edema: hypertension or increased intracranial pressure.
  - Migraines usually feel better after rest. If lasts >72 hours <u>not</u> usually a migraine.
  - Increased ICP headaches is exacerbated when lying down and need to consider hematomas or meningitis.

Treatment:

- The first preventative step is to avoid triggers (lifestyle modifications).
- First-line medications are NSAIDs or acetaminophen. Caffeine can be helpful.
- **Sumatriptans** (serotonin receptor <u>agonist</u>) used for acute management or if NSAIDs fail.

Prophylaxis: If >3 months use β-blockers (first-line prophylaxis), CCBs, or TCA.

Note: Coronary artery disease (CAD) needs to be ruled out before using sumatriptan; as it can cause vasoconstriction.

Cluster headache

Vascular etiology (extracranial vasodilation), lasts 30 minutes to 3 hours, and more common in males. Often associated with inheritance patterns and smokers.

Hx/PE: Usually present at night, periorbital headache, lacrimation, conjunctiva injections, nasal stuffiness, pain involves CN-V (V1 and V2 distribution).

Diagnosis:

- First time cluster headaches need consideration of further work-up to rule out:
  - Horner's syndrome: "PAM" ptosis, anhydrosis, and miosis (chest x-ray).
  - Giant cell (ESR levels and carotid Doppler).
  - Cavernous sinus infection (MRI scan with pituitary protocol).

Treatment:

- The first-line treatment is decrease exacerbation risk factors, such as alcohol intake, tobacco, and stressful exercise.
- Acute exacerbation: 100% oxygen and sumatriptan.

Prophylaxis:

- Transitional: prednisone.
- Maintenance: verapamil, lithium, or valproic acid.

Note: Beta-blockers are not useful for prophylaxis in cluster headaches.

Tension-type headache (stress headache)

Most common type of headache and possible association with neck and scalp muscle contractions and tension. Risk factors include increase fatigue and stress.

Hx/PE: More common in females, usually mild to moderate bilateral pain described as "band like," with pain localized in occipital or neck areas. No aura, audiophobia, nausea, or vomiting.

Diagnosis:

- Diagnosis of exclusion, if NSAIDs do not relieve the pain, then further work-up is required.
- ESR levels are needed in elderly patients to rule out giant cell.

Treatment:

- NSAIDs or acetaminophen (both first line).
- Sumatriptan (acute or severe).

Prophylaxis: TCAs, relaxation techniques, massages, and hot baths.

Cavernous sinus thrombosis (CST)

Occurs more commonly as a septic thrombosis (blood clot) in the cavernous sinus affecting cranial nerves II, III, IV, and VI; causing paralysis. Most common bacteria is secondary to *staphylococcus aureus* infection. CST can be life threatening and develop into sepsis or meningitis.

Hx/PE: Headache is the most common presentation, exophthalmos, and paralysis of cranial nerves. Patients with history of URI, sinusitis, or maxillary sinus infection can spread and develop into CST.

Diagnosis:

- CBC with L-shift, ESR, and blood culture (to rule out sepsis).
- Head MRI with pituitary protocol (gold standard).
- Lumbar puncture: if suspect meningitis.
- Source biopsy: if suspect fungal infection or patient has an atypical presentation.

Treatment:

- MSSA, then use nafcillin or oxacillin plus third-/fourth-generation cephalosporin plus metronidazole.
- MRSA, then use vancomycin plus third-/fourth-generation cephalosporin plus metronidazole.
- Place patient on thrombolytic therapy (controversial), if no contraindications are present.
- If not cured by antibiotics alone, may require surgical drainage. Sphenoidotomy can be indicated if the primary site of infection is the sphenoidal sinuses.

Note:

- ✓ Antibiotic use decreases incidence and mortality in CST.
- ✓ Rule out orbital cellulitis with CST.

Seizures

Common causes "VITAMINS" vascular, infection, trauma, autoimmune, metabolic, idiopathic, neoplastic, and sympathetic.

Risks of **Todd's paralysis** (post-seizure treatment): <u>unilateral</u> paralysis after seizure, which is usually intermittent.

<u>Precautions not acceptable during seizures</u>:

- Do not place things in patient's mouth during seizure.
- Do not restrain the patient.
- Do not call the ambulance unless seizure lasts more than 5–10 minutes.

Acceptable precautions during seizure:
- Place patient on side.
- Place soft object under patient's head.

Fun Facts:

- First time seizures are usually left untreated and will often require a work-up (unless simple febrile seizure); keep in mind that patients have a high risk of aspiration pneumonia and head hemorrhages.

- Treat first time seizures if there is a strong family history, abnormal EEG, or underlying pathology such as a tumor.

- Will not need work-up with EEG, unless there is <u>no</u> evidence of pathology from standard laboratory studies: CBC, electrolytes, glucose, ESR, TSH, calcium, ABG, EKG, UA, liver enzymes, blood alcohol levels, and toxicology screening (i.e., standard labs are the first orders, followed by EEG if labs are negative).

Partial seizures

Discrete region or epileptogenic focus. Both types of seizures usually last from about 30 seconds to 2 minutes. The brain has two hemispheres and each hemisphere has four lobes.

<u>Types</u>:

➤ **Simple partial seizure**: Affects a smaller part of one of the lobes. <u>No</u> loss of consciousness. Seizures can have psychic-like or dream-like features (hallucinations, déjà vu, fear, or postictal confusion).

➤ **Complex partial seizure:** Affects a larger part of the lobe or hemisphere. <u>Loss</u> of consciousness, motor, and sensory function. Presents with psychic features (hallucinations, déjà vu, fear, and postictal confusion).

Diagnosis:
- Order standard labs: CBC, electrolytes, glucose, ANA, TSH, EKG, ABG, ionized calcium, LFT, urinalysis, ESR, CRP, blood alcohol levels, and urine toxicology screening.

- EEG (gold standard, use when no confirmation with previous studies).

- Head MRI or head CT scan. Order with and without contrast to rule out neoplastic processes.

Treatment:
- First, treat the underlying causes.

- If recurrent partial or complex seizure: Phenytoin (first line), carbamazepine (Tegretol, only offered orally), or valproic acid.

- Children: if active seizure, use benzodiazepines as the first line medication; followed by barbiturates as the second line medication.

- Intractable temporal lobe seizures: **Temporal lobectomy** (definitive) after standard treatment has failed.

Tonic-clonic seizures (grand mal)

Usually idiopathic and effects the entire brain (both hemispheres), unlike partial seizures. Tonic-clonic seizures can evolve from partial seizures and can be associated with epilepsy.

Hx/PE: Loss of consciousness, symmetric tonic-clonic movements, incontinence, tongue biting, and postictal period.

Diagnosis:

- Rule out common causes with standard labs: CBC, electrolytes, ionized calcium, glucose, ESR, CRP, ABG, urinalysis, TSH, EKG, blood alcohol levels, and urine toxicology.
- EEG: "**10-Hz fast and slow waves**."
- Head MRI (order when underlying pathology is suspected).

Treatment:

- ABCs (always first step), treat underlying causes, and administer lorazepam or diazepam (if active seizure).
- Phenytoin or valproic acid (either is first-line therapy for long-term treatment).
- Keep in mind that most first-time seizures do <u>not</u> need treatment but do need work-up with standard labs. However, treatment should be started after first seizure if abnormal EEG, positive family history, or underlying pathology such as a brain tumor.
  - For example, if there is a brain tumor causing increased ICP, give steroids for acute relief.

<u>Anti-seizure medications</u>:

Phenytoin (Dilantin):

- ➤ In cases of continued seizures, measure phenytoin levels to determine whether within therapeutic index.
- ➤ Phenytoin needs to be tapered and <u>not</u> stopped abruptly; rather, dosages are decreased over time.

Side effects: can cause **gingival hypertrophy**, ataxia, slurred speech, confusion, nystagmus, double vision, and neuropathy.

Contraindicated in pregnancy causing **fetal hydantoin syndrome** (broad nasal bridge, wide fontanelle, cleft lip, cleft palate, microcephaly, low-set ears, absence of nails, and hypoplasia of distal phalanges).

Note: If toxic levels of phenytoin need to first decrease the dosage (do not stop medication abruptly).

Carbamazepine:

Used for seizures and neuropathic pain.

Side effects: can cause aplastic anemia (rare) and agranulocytosis (rare), and teratogenic (spina bifida).

Valproic acid: Teratogenic (do not switch or discontinue if already confirmed pregnancy but do switch regimen before pregnancy or planed pregnancy). Need to check alpha-fetoprotein. Breastfeeding is not usually contraindicated.

Absence seizures (petit mal)

A sudden brief loss and return of consciousness with no noticeable postictal state. Can be familial and more common in children. Seizures can last 5–10 seconds and can occur hundreds of times a day.

Hx/PE: Patient can appear to be daydreaming or staring, eye fluttering, and/or lip smacking. Can have impaired consciousness and good muscular tone.

Diagnosis:

- CBC, electrolytes, calcium, magnesium, glucose, urinalysis, TSH, ABG, liver enzymes, EEG, and MRI.
- EEG: "**classic three-per-second spike-and-wave**" or results can also be normal.

Treatment:

- First line treatment for acute seizures is stabilization and lorazepam or diazepam (rectally).

- Second line treatment for <u>acute</u> seizures is barbiturates, if benzodiazepines fail.
- **Ethosuximide** (first choice for <u>long-term</u> treatment) works by blocking low voltage T-type calcium channels.

Note: Absence seizures commonly diminish with age.

Status epilepticus

Medical emergency

Can be associated with anticonvulsant withdrawal, noncompliance with medications, anoxic brain injury, alcohol, infection, trauma, and drugs. Death can occur in 10%-30% of patients within 30 days.

Hx/PE: Defined as >5 minutes of repetitive seizures <u>or</u> greater than one seizures within 5 minutes, without returning to baseline consciousness.

Diagnosis:
- First ABCs (medical emergency).
- Order: CBC, electrolytes, glucose, ionized calcium, LFT, urinalysis, rhabdomyolysis, ABG, EKG, blood alcohol levels, and urine toxicology.
- Then, EEG and head MRI.
- If head trauma, have a low threshold for ordering a head CT scan.
- High risk of aspiration pneumonia (order chest x-ray).
- Rhabdomyolysis is common; be aware of acute renal failure (measure BUN/Cr ratio and CPK).

Note: An elevated prolactin level is consistent with epileptic seizure in the postictal period (specific).

Treatment:
- ABCs before obtaining labs.
- First medication is IV lorazepam (reassessment in 1 minute; if still seizing, then give a second dose of lorazepam with a loading dose of fosphenytoin or phenytoin).

- If continued seizure, intubate and administer IV phenobarbital.
- Start propofol if seizing persists.
- A cocktail of thiamine, glucose, and naloxone is commonly given.

Note: With seizures need to consider head injuries, shoulder dislocations, rhabdomyolysis, and aspiration pneumonia.

Infantile spasms (West syndrome)

Generalized epilepsy typically begins within the first 6 months of birth. Psychomotor development arrest and mental retardation are common. Highly associated with underlying central nervous system disorders.

<u>Risk factors:</u> Idiopathic or secondary to PKU, tuberous sclerosis, or hypoxic-ischemic injury.

Hx/PE: Jerking of the head, trunk, and extremities. Spasms will eventually decrease over time but the patient will continue with residual neurological impairment.

Diagnosis: Order: CBC, electrolytes, calcium, magnesium, ammonium levels, glucose, TSH, UA, LFTs, head MRI or head CT scan, lumbar puncture, and EEG: "**Hypsarrhythmia**" (high-voltage slow waves).

Treatment: First-line treatment: ACTH, prednisone, or valproic acid. West syndrome is very difficult to treat.

Vertigo/dizziness

Vertigo

Patient presents with the feeling of dizziness, spinning, or moving when they are not. They can also complain of nausea, vomiting, and ataxia.

<u>Types</u>:

➢ **Peripheral vertigo** (acute): Treat symptoms.

➤ Central vertigo (chronic): Head MRI.

➤ Presyncope vertigo: Usually cardiogenic.

Note:

✓ Peripheral nystagmus is usually horizontal and goes away when the patient focuses.

✓ Central nystagmus can be vertical or horizontal but does not go away with focus; order head MRI.

Benign paroxysmal positional vertigo (BPPV)

A disorder of the inter-ear that presents with transient vertigo lasting <1 minute. A type of peripheral vertigo caused by an otolith (95% are located in the semicircular canals).

Hx/PE: Vertigo and nystagmus triggered by change in head position or movement. Nausea and vomiting are not common and are dependent on the strength of the vertigo.

Diagnosis:

- Dix-Hallpike maneuver: Vertigo and nystagmus (toward the affected side).

- If nystagmus is out of proportion, then look for central lesions.

Treatment:

- Epley maneuver (270-degree rotation from Dix-Hallpike).

- Meclizine (anti-histamine) or scopolamine can be helpful for motion sickness and nausea.

Vestibular/cochlear pathology

Acute peripheral vestibulopathy

Secondary to acute inflammation of the vestibular (vertigo) or cochlear nerve (hearing loss). Common after a viral upper respiratory infection.

Hx/PE: Severe vertigo, nystagmus, gait abnormalities, nausea, and vomiting.

> ➤ **Labyrinthitis:** Hearing loss with auditory symptoms; mimics AICA stroke.
>   - Affects the *cochlear nerve* portion of CN VIII (tinnitus and hearing loss).
> ➤ **Vestibular neuritis:** <u>No</u> hearing loss with <u>no</u> auditory symptoms (tinnitus); mimics a PICA stroke.
>   - Affects the *vestibular nerve* portion of CN VIII (no hearing loss or tinnitus).
>   - Vestibular nerve (positive vertigo).

Diagnosis: **Vestibulo-ocular reflex.**

Treatment:

- Self-limited condition (usually spontaneously resolves within 1 month).
- <u>Acute</u>: Corticosteroids if given must be administered before 72 hours of symptoms.
- <u>Chronic</u>: Meclizine (vestibular sedative) helps with motion sickness.

Méniére's disease

Linked to elevated fluid levels in the inner ear, which can cause problems with hearing and balance. Has a similar presentation as labyrinthitis, however, Méniére's has a chronic course with relapse and remission.

Hx/PE: <u>Triad</u>: Tinnitus, fluctuating unilateral or bilateral hearing loss (<u>low</u> frequency), and severe vertigo. Most commonly unilateral and not all symptoms at the same time are required for diagnosis.

Diagnosis:

- Diagnosis of exclusion with at least two episodes lasting >20 minutes, with at least one abnormal audiometry.
- Audiogram and head MRI (rule out other pathologies).

- Sensorineural hearing loss: Perceive sound on normal ear.
- Conductive hearing loss: Perceive sound on affected ear.

Treatment:

- Acute exacerbation: Meclizine or scopolamine.
- Long-term treatment: Low-sodium diet (1-2 grams/day), diuretics, decrease caffeine intake and smoking.
- Severe disease: Surgery or gentamicin drops (aminoglycosides) to damage the vestibular nerve.

Toxic labyrinthitis

Present with vertigo and hearing loss often secondary to alcohol or medications such as aminoglycosides and cisplatin.

Diagnosis: Diagnosis of exclusion with suspicion of secondary medications.

Treatment: Remove the toxin.

Presbycusis

Bilateral sensorineural hearing loss; more common in aging adults with difficulty hearing high-frequency sounds. Most common cause of hearing loss in the elderly population.

Hx/PE: Can usually hear male voices better than females'. Voices become dull, difficulty using telephone, and difficulty discriminating against background noise. Look for a history of social withdrawal and isolation.

Diagnosis: **Hearing test** (with background noise) and otoscopy to rule out cerumen impaction.

Treatment: Hearing aids or cochlear implantation.

Otosclerosis

Genetic tendency by autosomal dominant inheritance, which causes progressive conductive or sensorineural hearing loss secondary to abnormal bone growth near the middle ear.

Hx/PE: Become clinically significant between ages 20 and 40. Hearing loss is usually bilateral, and symptoms often become worse during pregnancy or with OCP use.

Diagnosis: Otoscopy examination and audiometry.

Treatment:
- Sodium fluoride (slow progression of disease).
- Hearing aids (moderate).
- Removal of stapes bone (middle ear) **stapedectomy** with implantation and prosthesis (severe).

Neurological disorders

Myasthenia gravis

Autoimmune disease affecting anti-acetylcholine postsynaptic receptors that leads to progressive weakness that improves with rest (proximal muscles more affected than distal). Associated with thymomas (in 10% of cases) and other autoimmune disorders.

Myasthenia crisis: Respiratory compromise and aspiration pneumonia.

Hx/PE: Extraocular muscle weakness, ptosis (in at least 50% of patients), and intact reflexes.

Diagnosis:
- Best initial test: Measure **anti-acetylcholine receptor antibodies.**
- EMG under repetitive stimulation (most sensitive).
- Chest x-ray and chest CT scan to evaluate for thymoma (rule out lymphoma).

- Ice test for 5 minutes resolves ptosis (low cost and can provide helpful evidence).
- Edrophonium (<u>tensilon test</u>) is no longer used because of life-threating bradycardia.

Treatment:
- Best initial test: Pyridostigmine or neostigmine (acute symptomatic treatment).
    - Medications are acetylcholinesterase inhibitors.
- Prednisone (acute treatment) followed by azathioprine or cyclosporine (standard for long-term treatment).
- Plasmapheresis (severe) helps remove acetylcholine receptor antibodies.
- Surgical resection of thymoma is often curative.
- Myasthenic crisis: Treat with intubation first followed by plasmapheresis and IVIG, which are used for acute exacerbation.

Note: Avoid β-blockers and aminoglycosides, which can cause exacerbation. Also, avoid β-blockers in patients with psoriasis.

Lambert-Eaton myasthenic syndrome

Autoimmune disease affecting presynaptic voltage-gated calcium channels. Associated with small cell lung carcinoma of the lungs (in about 60% of cases).

Hx/PE: Proximal muscles, absent of DTRs, and muscle movements get better at the end of the day. Unlike myasthenia gravis, extraocular muscles and respiratory muscles are usually spared.

Diagnosis:
- EMG: "Incremental response" on repetitive nerve stimulation.
- Antibody to pre-synaptic calcium channels.
- Order: CPK (myositis) and TSH (thyroid dysfunction).
- Chest x-ray and chest CT scan to rule out small cell lung cancer.

Treatment:
- Pyridostigmine or neostigmine (improve neuromuscular transmission).

- Corticosteroids and immunosuppressants (azathioprine).
- Occasionally plasmapheresis and IVIG.
- If small cell lung cancer, treat with chemotherapy and/or radiation.

Trigeminal neuralgia

Also known as, tic douloureux; which is a chronic pain disease that affects the trigeminal nerve.

Hx/PE: Facial pain, facial spasms, and pain exacerbated by shaving or tooth brushing.

Diagnosis:
- Clinical diagnosis (tapping on the trigeminal nerve causes electric shock).
- Head MRI consideration to rule out MS or tumors.

Treatment:
- The first step is carbamazepine (anticonvulsants).
- If patient fails pharmaceutical treatment such as carbamazepine, the next step is surgical evaluation for decompressive surgery.

Note: Carbamazepine causes agranulocytosis and would be contraindicated in immunosuppressed patients.

Multiple sclerosis (MS)

An autoimmune disorder causing demyelination of the *myelin sheath* (protective covering of the nerves). More common in females and can be triggered by a viral infection and presents with "relapsing-remitting symptoms" separated by space and time.

Hx/PE: Optic neuritis (carries good prognosis), diplopia, weakness, urinary and bowel dysfunction (hypotonic bladder). Symptoms worsen after a hot shower. Can have an association with trigeminal neuralgias.

➤ Lhermitte sign: Electric shock-like pain that radiates down the spine with neck flexion; can be common in both MS and disc herniation.

➤ **Optic neuritis**: Painful visual loss (optic nerve), papilledema, and color loss. Fundoscopy may be normal (2/3) or with papillitis (1/3).

Diagnosis:
- The best diagnostic and most accurate test is a head MRI with gadolinium: Multiple asymmetric periventricular white matter lesions (**Dawson's fingers**).
- If head MRI findings are not conclusive, then obtain CSF sample to test for increased IgG, IgA, and IgM (**oligoclonal bands**), which are observed in 80–90% of patients.

Treatment:
- Corticosteroids (acute flares) with a high dose of IV methylprednisolone.
- INF-β1a, INF-β1b, or compolyer-1 (decreases relapse and delays disability onset).
- Mitoxantrone (progressive MS).
- Plasma exchange/plasmapheresis (severe cases).

Other treatments: Spasticity (baclofen), urinary retention (bethanicol), urinary incontinence (oxybutynin), painful paresthesias (amitriptyline), and fatigue (amantadine).

Guillain-Barré syndrome

Rapidly progressive damage to the peripheral nervous system secondary to acute inflammatory demyelinating polyneuropathy; usually after GI infection with *Campylobacter* or viral infection. Approximately 85% of patients make a complete recovery.

Hx/PE: Neuropathy (numbness, tingling, and pain) starts distally and progresses proximally "ascending paralysis." Advanced stages may present with hyporeflexia and affected respiratory muscles. The disease can progress fast and may necessitate ICU care.

Diagnosis:
- CSF (initial diagnostic study) testing for **albuminocytologic dissociation.**

- EMG (most sensitive and confirms diagnosis) shows decreased nerve conduction.
- Stool culture can be helpful.
- Vital capacity is the best indication of respiratory status.

Treatment:

- Plasmapheresis and IVIG (both equally effective and first line).
- All patients should be hospitalized regardless of disease severity.
- Have a very low threshold for ICU admission and intubation (respiratory failure, aspiration risk, or rapid deceleration).
- Will need physical therapy, occupational therapy, and speech therapy.

Note: Never give glucocorticoid steroids to these patients (delays recovery).

Amyotrophic lateral sclerosis (Lou Gehrig's)

Chronic slow progression of cell death in *lateral corticospinal tracts* (upper and lower motor loss). Patient feeling trapped in one's body, have normal intelligence, normal bowel and urinary function, and intact sensory function.

➤ Damage of upper motor neurons: Spasticity and increased DTRs.

➤ Damage of lower motor neurons: Flaccidity, weakness, and atrophy.

Diagnosis:

- Clinical presentation.
- EMG (widespread denervation) and PFTs (is very important in ALS).
- Cervical spine MRI to rule out structural lesions or tumors.

Treatment:

- Supportive treatment.
- **Riluzole** (slows progression, which increases survival).

- Consider aspiration precautions, respiratory dysfunction (tracheostomy) and percutaneous gastrostomy tubes (PEG) when patients present with dysphagia (non-reversible).
- Will need physical therapy, occupational therapy, speech therapy, and nutritional support.
- Death usually occurs 3–5 years after diagnosis from respiratory failure (diaphragmatic paralysis).

Dementia

Alzheimer's disease

Gradual neurodegenerative disease that causes short-term memory loss first (anterograde first followed by retrograde), personality intact at first, more common in females, family history, "neurofibrillary tangles," neurotic plaques with amyloid deposits, amnesia, and high risk of aspiration pneumonia (commonly the cause of death). Alzheimer's disease is the most common cause of dementia.

Diagnosis:
- The first step in diagnosis is to conduct a MMSE and is essentially a clinical diagnosis (need to have memory loss with executive function loss).
- Always rule out depression, vitamin B12, VDRL (usually if high risk), TSH, free T4, and glucose.
- Brain MRI: can show cortical atrophy (rule out age-appropriate atrophy).
- PET scan: Temporoparietal hypometabolism.
- Autopsy provides a definitive diagnosis but is rarely done.

Note: Noncontrast head CT scan or MRI scan is recommended to rule out structural abnormalities in subjects with dementia. A specific **apolipoprotein E gene** allele is associated with Alzheimer's dementia, but testing is controversial.

Treatment:
- Supportive treatment.

- Vitamin E and Ginkgo biloba have modest efficacy.
- Treatments of choice for Alzheimer's disease: **Donepezil**, galantamine, or rivastigmine have been shown to slow decline and improve cognitive function → acetylcholinesterase inhibitor.
- **Memantine**: (Linked to learning and memory) → NMDA receptor antagonist.
    - Can use memantine for moderate Alzheimer's.
    - Memantine has little effect on the treatment of mild Alzheimer's disease.
- If paranoid delusion and agitation develops, a low dose of atypical antipsychotic medication can be started.
- Tacrine can cause liver toxicity and is rarely used.

Note:

✓ Medications only slow progression but do not cure the disease.

✓ Have a low threshold for placing patient on aspiration precautions.

Vascular dementia

Vascular dementia is caused by multiple minor ischemic strokes that causes an <u>abrupt</u> onset with "step-wise" memory degradation and possible focal neurological findings.

<u>Risks factors</u> are the same as those for strokes.

Diagnosis:

- The first step is head CT scan w/o contrast to rule out hemorrhage, followed by head MRI to reveal old infarcts.
- Order similar labs, as for ischemic strokes: PTT, PT/INR, platelets, EKG, echocardiogram, carotid Doppler, and lipid profile.
- Need to rule out vitamin B12, VDRL, finger stick glucose, TSH, and depression.

Treatment:

- The Food and Drug Administration (FDA) have not approved any drugs specifically to treat vascular dementia but controlling risk factors such as, blood pressure, hyperlipidemia, diabetes, exercise, and weight loss can be helpful.

- Donepezil, memantine, vitamin E, and ginkgo biloba; have been shown to have small benefits.

Note: Head MRI is more specific than head CT scan for ischemia strokes.

Pick's disease

A neurodegenerative disease that causes frontotemperal dementia.

Hx/PE: Personality changes and compulsive behaviors are the first changes. Can present with impulsivity, repetitive behaviors, hypersexuality, and hyperorality. <u>No</u> movement disorder.

Diagnosis:

- First order vitamin B12, fasting glucose, VDRL, and TSH.
- Head MRI (frontal and temporal atrophy) and **Pick bodies** (on biopsy).

Treatment:

- No curative therapy but behavior management is helpful.
- Can place patient on same medications as Alzheimer's disease but will have less overall response.

Note: Consider urine toxicology screening in patients with AMS.

AIDS dementia

Cognitive impairment, incontinence, motor skill impairment, and confusion. Need to exclude other pathologies first.

Diagnosis:

- In cases of acute dementia and delirium, vital signs and basic laboratory data should always be checked first (B12, VDRL, TSH, glucose, and depression).
- Diagnosis of exclusion → measure CD4+ and viral load.

- Head MRI (may show cortical and subcortical brain atrophy).
- Lumbar puncture findings can be normal.

Treatment: Antiviral medication (HARRT).

Normal pressure hydrocephalus (NPH)

An elevated level of CSF in the brain, in which the fluid most commonly accumulates in the ventricles and can cause pressure gradients of 150 to 200 mm H_2O.

Hx/PE: "Wet-wobbly and wacky" urinary incontinence, abnormal gait, and dementia. Signs of increased ICP like papilledema do not appear. Gait is described as "glued to the floor."

Diagnosis:
- Head CT scan without contrast (ventricular enlargement).
- Lumbar puncture (elevated pressure).

Treatment:
- Large-volume lumbar puncture (30–50 mL) is the gold standard.
- Lumbar puncture improves symptoms.
- Long-term treatment involves shunt placement.

Note:
- ✓If urinary incontinence needs to rule out consider DM, SIADH, and UTI.
- ✓Dementia rule out B12, VDRL, glucose, TSH, and depression.
- ✓Lumbar puncture for NPH is both diagnostic and therapeutic.

Creutzfeldt–Jakob disease

Also known as spongiform encephalopathies, this disease is characterized by prions, spongy degeneration, neuronal loss, subacute dementia, myoclonic jerks, and rapid dementia onset within weeks to months.

- Head MRI (increased T2 and FLAIR intensity).
- EEG (pyramidal signs and periodic <u>sharp</u> waves).
- CSF (normal or 14-3-3 proteins).
- Autopsy (definitive and more accurate diagnosis).

Treatment: No effective treatment.

Movement disorders

Huntington's disease (HD)

Autosomal dominant (50% chance of passing to offspring) disease that affects muscle coordination; caused by an expansion of a CAG triple repeat on the short arm of chromosome 4 in the *HD* gene. Carries risk of anticipation, which causes younger onset in subsequent generations.

Hx/PE: Gradual onset, **chorea** (sudden onset of purposeless "dance-like" movements), altered behaviors, dementia, antisocial behavior, and irritability.

Diagnosis:

- Specific genetic testing (best test).
- Head MRI: Cerebral atrophy especially the caudate and putamen and lateral ventricle widening.

Treatment:

- No direct cure but can consider treating depression and psychotic symptoms.
- Antipsychotics (symptomatic control) or **tetrabenazine** (movement disorder) are used to treat choreiform and chorea movements.
- Multiple discipline: Physical therapy, occupational therapy, speech therapy, and genetic counseling.

Note:

✓Encourage the patient to disclose test results to family for support. If they refuse, document interaction in their chart.

✓Tetrabenazine can be used for other movement disorders such as HD, Tourette syndrome, and tardive dyskinesia.

Parkinson's disease

A central nervous system disease affect primarily the muscular system. Decreased dopamine and increased acetylcholine levels. Often associated with dementia and depression during advanced stages.

Hx/PE: Triad: Resting tremor ("**pill rolling**"), bradykinesia (slow movements), and rigidity ("**cogwheeling**"). Other associated symptoms are masked facies, memory loss, and stooped posture.

Types of gait:

➢ **Cerebral ataxia**: "Drunken sailor" noted as zigzagging.

➢ **Senile gait**: "Walking on ice" characterized by slow careful movements.

➢ **Shuffling gait**: "Decreased speed and amplitude."

Diagnosis:

- Clinical diagnosis that requires bradykinesia, with tremor or rigidity.
- Rule out other pathologies such as MPTP, manganese, neuroleptic medications, and thyroid dysfunction (TSH and free T4).

Treatment:

- Mild disease: Ropinirole, bromocriptine, and pramipexole (partial dopamine agonists).
- Mild disease and <60 years: Trihexyphenidyl (anticholinergic agents).
- Mild disease >60 years: Amantadine.
- Moderate/severe disease: Levodopa and carbidopa.
- Selegiline: (MAO-B) → helps arrest progression.
- If medical therapy fails, consider surgical **pallidotomy** or **deep brain stimulation**.

Note:

- ✓ Trihexyphenidyl side effects: "Dry as a bone, red as a beet, and mad as a hatter." Patients <60 years can better handle the possible side effects.
- ✓ Always consider SSRIs for depression in patients with Parkinson's disease.
- ✓ If a patient develops psychosis while on a dopamine agonist, consider antipsychotic use rather than medication discontinuation.

Essential tremor

The cause of essential tremor is unknown but appears to be familial. Is often described as an action tremor.

Hx/PE: Tremor worse with movement ("intentional tremor") and improves with rest and alcohol intake. Patients have a normal life expectancy.

Diagnosis: Clinical diagnosis (presents of action tremor); no need for head MRI scan.

Treatment:

- β-blockers (propranolol) are the treatment of choice.
- If a patient has bradycardia, asthma, or COPD, then use **primidone** (anti-epileptic) or benzodiazepine.
- When conservative medication are not helpful, consider botulinum toxin or deep brain stimulation.

Note: Avoid caffeine and stress with essential tremor.

Brain neoplasms

➤ Approximately 40% are benign and rarely metastasize; however, brain metastases are most commonly from lung cancers.

➢ Metastases usually occur at the gray and white matter junction.

➢ Metastatic malignant disease is more common than primary malignancy in the brain. The treatment is whole-brain radiation therapy to increase survival and help alleviate pain.

Hx/PE: Brain neoplasms can cause seizures and focal motor deficits; only ~30% of patients experience headaches. Headaches are classically worse in the mornings.

Other common cancer metastases and locations:

■ Gastrointestinal adenocarcinoma usually metastasizes to the liver then lungs.

■ Prostate cancer usually goes first to lymph nodes then lung and/or bone.

Types of brain tumors:

➢ **Astrocytoma**: Most common brain tumor in children; associated with GFAP overexpression.

➢ **Medulloblastoma**: Second most common in children. They arise in the cerebellar vermis and grow down into the fourth ventricle. Can cause truncal ataxia and unsteady gait. Primitive neuroectodermal tumor (PNET), hydrocephalus, and increased ICP.

➢ **Hemangioblastoma**: Benign tumor with a prominent capillary network. The cerebellar hemispheres are the most common locations. Associated with von Hippel-Lindau syndrome.

➢ **Oligodendroglioma**: Composed of neoplastic oligodendroglial cells. Usually arises in the cerebral white matter.

➢ **Glioblastoma multiforme**: (Grade IV astrocytoma): Most common in adults, high mitotic activity, and can cause extensive necrosis and hemorrhage within the tumor. "**Butterfly pattern**," crosses the corpus callosum, and characterized by a ring-enhancing lesion on head MRI. Other conditions with ring-enhancing lesions on radiologic studies are toxoplasmosis and CNS lymphomas.

➢ **Meningioma**: Derived from meningothelial cells and appear as dural-attached masses.

➢ **Acoustic neuroma (schwannoma):** Arises from Schwann cells; characterized by unilateral hearing loss, tinnitus, and vertigo. Need to rule out Méniére's disease. Associated with neurofibromatosis (NF) and von Recklinghausen's disease.

➤ **Ependymoma**: Has an ependymal origin and grows as a mass that fills the fourth ventricle. Can cause obstructive hydrocephalus and increase ICP.

➤ **Craniopharyngioma**: Occurs in the suprasellar region and produces endocrine symptoms such as panhypopituitarism. Presence of bitemporal hemianopsia involving the optic chiasm and calcification above the sella on neuroimaging.

➤ **Pinealoma**: **Parinaud's sign** (vertical gaze paralysis).

Diagnosis:

- First test is a head CT scan <u>with</u> contrast (good for assessing hydrocephalus or when MRI is not available).
- Gadolinium-enhanced head MRI (appropriate for soft tissue).
- Biopsy with a CT-guided biopsy and debulking if necessary.
- Need to perform CT/MRI scanning prior to lumbar puncture, which can cause herniation.

Note: Lumbar puncture can cause herniation if patient has brain tumors, brain abscesses, and hydrocephalus.

Treatment:

- Surgical resection (if possible), whole-brain radiation, and chemotherapy.
  - Brain cancers rarely metastasize because of blood-brain barrier, so chemotherapy is rarely used.
- Corticosteroids or shunts, can be used to decrease ICP.
- Consider seizure prophylaxis.

Pseudotumor cerebri

Also known as **idiopathic intracranial hypertension**; classically occurs in obese young females of childbearing age on OCPs, taking tetracycline antibiotics, or high-dose vitamin A.

Hx/PE: Headaches worse in the morning and exacerbated by coughing and sneezing. Presents with papilledema (primary physical finding), <u>no</u> nuchal rigidity, <u>no</u> Kerning sign, and <u>no</u> Brudzinski sign.

- Head MRI/CT scan: Normal but needed to rule out other causes.
- Lumbar puncture: Measure open pressure (elevated).

Treatment:

- Weight loss and discontinue OCPs.
- Lumbar puncture and acetazolamide (decreases CSF production).
- Venous sinus stenting.
- The most important goal is to preserve vision.

Note: Mannitol decreases cerebral edema but does not decrease CSF production (like acetazolamide).

Arnold-Chiari malformation

Arnold-Chiari malformation II: A congenital disorder that results in displacement of the cerebellar hemispheres and medulla through the foramen magnum. Commonly associated with **syringomyelia** that presents with bilateral loss of pain and temperature sensation at the <u>level</u> of the lesion.

Diagnosis: Neuroimaging with MRI is the best imaging modality.

Treatment: No current cure, the treatments is based on surgery and management of symptoms.

Neurocutaneous disorders

Neurofibromatosis (NF)

Autosomal dominant. A tumor disorder that is caused by a mutation of chromosome 17. Can cause neurofibroms, scoliosis, dermatological manifestations, learning disabilities, vision disorders, and seizures.

Types:

➤ **NF type I:** (Chromosome 17).

➤ **NF type II:** (Chromosome 22).

Hx/PE: "**Café-au-lait spots**," neurofibromas, freckling, optic glioma, seizures, skin nodules, and pheochromocytoma. NF type II (bilateral acoustic neuromas).

Diagnosis:

- Head MRI with gadolinium.
- Genetic testing: NF-I (chromosome 17) and NF-II (chromosome 22).
- Need to complete dermatologic, ophthalmologic, and auditory testing.

Treatment: No cure but can treat underlying diseases such as acoustic neuromas and optic gliomas (surgery and/or radiosurgery).

Tuberous sclerosis

Autosomal dominant, multiple systemic, seizures, "**ash-leaf**" hypopigmented lesions, mental retardation, sebaceous adenomas, cardiac rhabdomyomas, and renal hamartomas. Look out for infantile spasms and thick hypopigmented lesions.

Diagnosis:

- Skin lesions: Wood's UV lamp.
- Head CT scan: Malignant astrocytomas.
- EKG: Rhabdomyomas of the heart.
- Renal ultrasound: Renal hamartomas or polycystic disease.
- Renal CT scan: Angiomyolipomas.
- Chest X-ray: Pulmonary lesions or cardiomegaly secondary to rhabdomyomas.

Treatment:

- Adenoma sebaceum: Cosmetic surgery.
- Seizures: Phenytoin.
- Infantile spasms: ACTH and/or prednisone.

Aphasias

Broca's aphasia

Also known as **expressive aphasia**. Affects the language production area particularly the *inferior frontal gyrus* (brodmann areas 44 and 45), causing motor aphasia and awareness disorder, and is most commonly associated to MCA stroke.

Hx/PE: Impaired speech, frustration with awareness of dysfunction, hemiparesis, and hemisensory loss in the upper extremities and face. Patients are agrammatical with frequent pauses and often use word substitution.

Treatment:
- Speech therapy.
- Some studies have shown that **piracetam** (a cyclic derivative of GABA) and amphetamines can be helpful.

Wernicke's aphasia

Also known as, **receptive aphasia**. Affects the language comprehension area, *superior temporal gyrus* (brodmann area 22), and sensory aphasia.

Hx/PE: The patient is <u>unaware</u> of aphasia and has poor understanding of spoken speech. They may have preserved fluency but with "**word salad**." Commonly associated with MCA stroke.

Treatment: Speech therapy.

Comas

Profound suppression of responses to internal and external stimuli (unarousable and unresponsive). Coma indicates bilateral dysfunction of both cerebral hemispheres at the level of the pons or higher.

Lesser states: Obtundation or stupor.

Common causes: Stroke, hypoxia, hypoglycemia, hypothermia, hyperthermia, hemorrhage, axonal injury infection, seiz ure, thiamine deficiency, thyroid dysfunction, diffuse ischemic encephalopathy, and toxin exposure.

Diagnosis:
- First step is ABCs.
- Monitor vital signs, temperature, Glasgow coma scale, corneal reflex, gag reflex, and oculocephalic reflex.
- Physical exam: Neurological exam (CNs, sensory, motor, DTR, and cerebellar).
- Common labs: CBC, CMP, glucose, NH3, TSH, free T4, EKG, D-dimers, ABG, ESR, urine toxicology screening, blood alcohol levels, head CT scan, head MRI, LP, and EEG.

Treatment: First ABCs and medical cocktail (if unknown etiology): "**DONT**" dextrose, O2, naloxone, and thymine. Place on cardiorespiratory monitoring. Treat underlying causes.

Types of comas:
- **Locked-in-syndrome.** Wakeful and alert, spontaneously opens eyes and spontaneous respiration drive.
  An example is advanced ALS.
- **Persistent vegetative state.** Wakefulness without awareness and with spontaneous respiration drive. An example is anoxic brain injury.
- **Coma.** Unconscious, no sleep–wake cycles, and spontaneous respiration.
- **Brain death.** Unconscious, no sleep–wake cycles, and no spontaneousrespiration.

Note: All patients with AMS with unknown etiology should receive oxygen, dextrose, thiamine, and naloxone. Also, need to check blood alcohol levels and urine toxicology.

Wernicke's and Korsakoff's

Wernicke's encephalopathy

Medical emergency

Involves lack of thiamine (an essential coenzyme in carbohydrate metabolism) in the brain, more commonly effecting the mammillary bodies and thalamus. Common in alcoholics, starvation, AIDS, and high glucose levels. This is a <u>reversible</u> disease.

Hx/PE: <u>Triad</u>: Encephalopathy (global brain dysfunction), ophthalmoplegia (weakness or paralysis of one or more of the extraocular muscles), and ataxia.

Diagnosis: If memory loss order: Glucose levels, B12 levels, VDRL, TSH, blood alcohol levels, toxicology screening, and head CT scan (if needed).

Treatment:

- Give IV <u>or</u> IM thiamine and magnesium sulfate before glucose; decreases the risk of Wernicke encephalopathy exacerbation due to high glucose metabolism in the brain.
- When stabilized switch IV thiamine to oral thiamine.
- Other common deficient vitamins are folic acid and B12.

Note: Glucose given before thiamine can exacerbate thiamine deficiency.

Korsakoff's dementia

Almost exclusively found in alcoholics and is caused by low levels of thiamine in the brain.

Hx/PE: <u>Triad</u>: Encephalopathy, ophthalmoplegia, ataxia, and anterograde/retrograde memory loss. Add confabulations, horizontal nystagmus, and <u>irreversible</u> disease.

Diagnosis: If memory loss order: Glucose levels, B12 levels, VDRL, TSH, blood alcohol levels, toxicology screening, and head CT scan (if needed).

Treatment: Thiamine before glucose, magnesium sulfate, folic acid, and B12.

Vitamin B12 deficiency (subacute combined degeneration)

Deficient levels of vitamin B12 can cause degeneration of many combined CNS regions, megaloblastic anemia, peripheral neuropathy (numbness, tingling, and pain), symmetric stocking-glove sensory and motor neuropathy, bowel and bladder dysfunction, and delirium/dementia.

<u>Risk factors</u>: "Strict vegetarians," post gastric or ileal resection, pernicious anemia, Crohn's disease, alcoholism, and malnutrition.

Diagnosis:

- First step, order CBC with peripheral blood smear followed by MCV (macrocytic cells).
  - CBC (anemia) with peripheral blood smear (hypersegmented neutrophils).
- Measure B12 levels (low) and MMA (elevated).
  - Order MMA, if normal B12 levels with high suspicion.
- MMA (elevated) is specific for B12 and rules out folic acid deficiency.
- Reticulocyte levels are low in B12 deficiency.
  - Reticulocytes are the first laboratory results to become elevated with B12 replacement.

Treatment: Replace vitamin B12 orally or IV. Can have good prognosis and complete recovery of both anemia and peripheral neuropathy.

Note:

✓B12 levels can be falsely normal in about one-third of patients.

This is why diagnosis is contingent on peripheral blood smear results.

✓ Patients need to be monitored during treatment with B12, as replacement can lead to hypokalemia.

Folate deficiency

Deficient levels of folic acid (vitamin B9) can cause megaloblastic anemia without neurological abnormalities.

<u>Risk factors:</u> Alcoholism, methotrexate, sulfa medications, malnutrition, and "meat lovers."

Diagnosis:

- First test, ordered CBC with peripheral blood smear (anemia and hypersegmented neutrophils), then order MCV (macrocytic).
- Measure folic acid (low), MMA (normal), and homocysteine (elevated).
    - Order homocysteine levels, if normal folic acid levels with high suspicion.

Treatment: Replace with oral or IV folic acid.

Ocular pathology

Closed-angle glaucoma

Medical emergency

Usually caused by elevated ocular pressure, which leads to damage of the optic nerve (visual loss). When the iris dilates, it pushes against the lens and causes fluid to remain in the posterior chamber. More common in Asian populations.

Hx/PE: Unilateral eye pain accompanied by headache, blurred vision, and "peripheral vision loss." The patient may present with slightly dilated pupils.

Diagnosis:

- Clinical diagnosis with symptoms worse at night or after watching a movie in the dark.
- Snellen chart and tonometry (IOP test, >30 mmHg).

Treatment:

- **Medical emergency**.
- The first medication given should be <u>topical</u> pilocarpine eye drops; decreases IOP and the risk of blindness.
- Medications include timolol (lowers the amount of fluid), pilocarpine (opens the angle to allow drainage), oral or IV acetazolamide (reduces fluid), and IV mannitol.
- <u>Severe</u>: **Laser peripheral iridotomy**.

Note: Aqueous humor is produced in the **ciliary body** of the iris and drains via the **trabecular meshwork**.

Open-angle glaucoma

The aqueous humor through the trabecular meshwork is limited, which causes elevation in the aqueous pressure. Common in African Americans and results in frequent change in lens strength. Most common glaucoma in the United States.

Hx/PE: Headaches, visual disturbances, blurry vision, peripheral vision loss, seeing "halos" around objects, and progressive visual loss.

Diagnosis:

- Visual field testing (Snellen test).
- **Tonometry** (measures increased pressure, >30 mmHg).
- Ophthalmoscopy (optic nerve cupping).

Treatment:

- Timolol (decreased aqueous production), pilocarpine (increased aqueous outflow), and acetazolamide (reduces fluid).
- <u>Severe</u>: **Laser trabeculoplasty** or **laser trabeculectomy**.

Note: Caffeine can cause elevation of IOP in patients with glaucoma.

Age-related macular degeneration

Most common cause of <u>bilateral</u> blindness in the United States, in the elderly population (strongest predictor). Loss of central vision (the macula) because of damage to the retina. Can be associated with cataracts.

<u>Types</u>:

➤ **Atrophic degeneration**: (Dry) caused by scaring and fibrosis, which leads to gradual visual loss.

➤ **Exudative/neovascular degeneration**: (Wet) caused by neovascularization, which causes exudative fluid and more rapid visual loss.

Hx/PE: "Painless loss of <u>central</u> vision," difficult to read, and recognize faces. Peripheral vision intact.

Diagnosis: Funduscopic examination (Drusen spots), Amsler grid (wavy lines), Snellen test, and angiography (neovascularization).

- <u>Atrophic</u>: Drusen and/or pigmentary changes.
- <u>Exudative</u>: Subretinal fluid.

Treatment:

- <u>Atrophic</u>: No treatment. Vitamin C, vitamin E, beta-carotene, and zinc can be helpful.
- <u>Exudative</u>: Vascular endothelial growth factor (VEGF) inhibitors and photodynamic therapy with **verteporfin** (destroys vessels).

Central retinal artery occlusion

Thrombolysis of the ophthalmic artery. **Amaurosis fugax** (transient blindness) is an acute ischemia of the retinal artery. Associated with carotid artery atherosclerosis.

<u>Risk factors</u>: The same as for any thrombolysis.

Hx/PE: Sudden onset of painless <u>unilateral</u> blindness.

Diagnosis:

- Optic exam (fundoscopic examination) reveals diminished perfusion and "cherry-red" spot at the fovea.
- Often associated with carotid bruit (evaluate with carotid Doppler, lipids, echocardiogram, glucose levels, and blood pressure).

Treatment:

- Treatment is controversial and needs to be given within 2-4 hours:
  - Hyperbaric oxygen therapy or oxygen therapy with 5% carbon dioxide and 95% oxygen.
  - Other measures of increasing IOP, is by applying direct pressure on the eye or breathing in a paper bag.
  - Consider administering thrombolytics and/or IV acetazolamide.

Central retinal vein occlusion

Occlusion of the main vein in the retina, which causes fluid to collect in the macula (macular edema).

Hx/PE: Sudden painless <u>unilateral</u> visual loss.

Diagnosis: Fundoscopic examination "cotton-wool" spots, macular edema, disk swelling, venous dilation, and retinal hemorrhage. **Fluorescein angiography** can help visualize occlusion.

Treatment:

- No effective medical treatment for central retinal vein occlusion.
- Aspirin, anticoagulation, and laser photocoagulation have variable results.

Retinal detachment

Medical emergency

Caused by separation of the retina from underlying ocular tissue. Risk factors include trauma, opthalimic surgery, and sever myopia.

Hx/PE: <u>Painless</u> unilateral visual loss, presents with floaters (increased floaters equals worse prognosis), and blind spot. Patient reports the feeling of a "curtain falling" over their visual field.

Diagnosis: Can be examined by **fundus photography** or ophthalmoscopy.

Treatment: Medical emergency (call an ophthalmologist). Consider laser photocoagulation surgery or scleral buckle surgery.

Retro-orbital hematoma

Medical emergency

Most commonly secondary to facial/orbital trauma and can lead to acute orbital compartment syndrome.

Diagnosis: Head radiological studies and ophthalmoscopy.

Treatment: Immediate ophthalmologic consult.

Pterygium

Benign growth of vascularized conjunctivae that extends onto the cornea.

Diagnosis: Clinical diagnosis.

Treatment: Remove surgically (elective); no intervention is also appropriate (if asymptomatic).

<u>Prevention</u>: Wear protective sunglasses, minimized wind, and sun exposure.

Strabismus

Also known as "crossed eyes". Occurs when eyes do not line up in the same direction (eyes do not look at the same object at the same time). The cause is because the eye muscles do not work together to focus on one object.

Hx/PE: Eyes do not align in same direction and patient can complain of double vision.

Diagnosis: Corneal light test (pupils are asymmetric).

Treatment: Place eye patch on the dominant eye and surgery if this does not produce improvement.

Pseudostrabismus

Considered the false appearance of strabismus. Eyes appear to be crossed eyes, but usually due to abnormal facial features, such as wide nasal bridge. Common in East Asian infants because of epicanthic folds covering the medial aspect of the eyes.

Diagnosis: Corneal light test (pupils are symmetric).

Treatment: No treatment, as eyes are aligned normally.

Psychiatry

Pediatric psychiatry

Mental retardation

Must exhibit deficits in both intellectual and social adaptive functioning. More common in males.

Ranges:

- Average IQ: 100.
- Normal IQ: 70-100.
- Mild IQ: 50–70.
- Moderate IQ: 30–50.
- Severe IQ: 20–30.
- Profound IQ: below 20.

Diagnosis: Genetic testing and rule out secondary causes (CBC, electrolytes, TSH, FT4, fasting glucose, depression, B12 levels, urinalysis, and hearing test).

Treatment:

- *Patient's education*: special education, behavioral therapy, physical therapy, and speech therapy.
- P*arent's education*: genetic counseling and safe environment.

Rett syndrome

X-linked dominant disorder (gene MCPE2). More common in girls. Characteristics include seizures (80%), movement disorders, and sighing (which mimics autistic behavior). During the first 5 months infant has age-appropriate motor skills, head circumference, growth, and social interaction.

Hx/PE: Characteristic handwriting, speech loss, and psychomotor retardation (e.g., frequently place hands in mouth).

Diagnosis:

- Clinical diagnosis or genetic testing (confirmatory).
- Other test in evaluation: hearing test, visual testing, head CT-scan, and EEG.

Treatment:

- There is no cure and supportive measures need to be considered such as, family counseling, behavior therapy, special education, and physical therapy for muscular dysfunction.
- Control seizures (phenytoin), movement disorders, and self-harming behavior (anti-psychotics [D2-antagonist]).

Prognosis: life expectancy middle age and beyond.

Note: after 6 months of age, there is a decline in motor skills, social skills, loss of eye contact, and deceleration of head circumference, weight, and height.

Asperger's syndrome

More common in males. Pervasive developmental disorder, which differs from autism because patients are more communicative, social, and milder language impairment; however, they do struggle with these issues. They are more likely to present with impaired social interaction and repetitive behavior.

Hx/PE: Characteristics include abnormal social interactions, language, intellectual deficits, repetitive behavior, social impairments, poor motor coordination, and obsessional interests.

Diagnosis: Clinical diagnosis.

Treatment:

- No medications directly treats Asperger's disorder.
- Supportive care: improve relationships with others, occupational and physical therapy, speech therapy, special education, and behavioral therapy.

Childhood disintegrative disorder

A rare disorder more common in males, with a <u>delayed</u> onset of development in speech, motor, and social functioning.

Hx/PE: Normal development for the first 2 years then regression in functioning in domains such as language, social, motor, and bladder function. Also includes repetitive behaviors.

Diagnosis: Clinical diagnosis and need to rule out, genetic testing, CBC, electrolytes, TSH, glucose, B12, hearing test, visual testing, head CT scan, and EEG.

Treatment: Family counseling, behavior therapy, special education, speech therapy, and antipsychotics (if aggression or harm to self). Anticonvulsant medications are used to control seizures.

Autistic disorder

More common in males. Developmental disorder including impaired social interaction, verbal and nonverbal communication deficits, and irregular responses to the environment. Usually develops by 3 years of age.

Hx/PE: Delay or absence of smiling in social situations, lack of eye contact, bizarre speech, banging of head, self-injury, decreased social interaction, stereotypical movements, and anger.

Diagnosis: Clinical diagnosis and rule out genetic testing, neuroimaging, metabolic profile, hearing test, and visual testing. Neuroimaging and metabolic profiles are not always routine but can be helpful.

Treatment:

- Family counseling, behavior therapy, special education, speech therapy, and improvement of social interactions.

- Medication considerations: anti-convulsants, anti-depressants, and anti-psychotics.

Note: development of interpersonal relationships is one of the most challenging obstacles for autistic patients.

Attention deficit hyperactive disorder (ADHD)

Symptoms must be present for at least 6 months with onset occurring between 6 months to 7 years of age. Needs to be present in at least <u>two</u> settings (e.g., home and school). Children have normal intelligence.

<u>Risks</u>: have a greater risk than general population for developing conduct disorder and antisocial personality disorder.

Hx/PE: Inattention, short attention span, or hyperactivity.

Diagnosis:

- ADHD is over diagnosed and necessary to rule out **normal child behavior**.

- ADHD symptoms are estimated to decline by 50% every 5 years until the mid-20s and can persist into adulthood for 30% of patients.

Treatment:

- *First-line treatment* is stability (behavioral therapy), structure at home, and school.

- If first-line treatment fails, then initiate medications (**methylphenidate** or dextroamphetamine).

<u>Side effects of medications:</u> include insomnia, decreased appetite, weight loss, and headaches.

Note:

- ✓ Assessment of cardiac history and physical examination needs to be given before providing stimulant therapy. If cardiac history consideration of EKG and pediatric cardiologist consult.

✓ Stimulant therapy treatment for ADHD does not increase risk of substance disorders in this population.

✓ Beware that stimulants can be misused and abused. Monitor pervious history of ADHD.

Oppositional defiant disorder (ODD)

Must be present for at least *6 month* and interfere with social and academic performance. More common in males and patient needs to be <18 years of age before diagnosis.

Hx/PE: Argumentative, temper tantrums, and problems with authority figures.

Diagnosis: Clinical diagnosis by obtaining a good patient history.

Treatment: Behavior therapy, social skill training, and family therapy.

Conduct disorder

More common in males and need to be <18 years of age before diagnosis. More commonly found in children with parents who are antisocial or have alcohol dependence. Conduct disorder are more physically aggressive in comparison to ODD. Can be associated with ADHD and substance abuse.

Hx/PE: Shows defiance against laws or rules, aggression to others, cruelty to animals, fighting, or destruction of property.

Treatment:

- Behavioral intervention using rewards system.
- Multi-systemic intervention involving individual, family, and school.
- If aggressive, antipsychotics may be useful.

Note:

✓ Patients can be charming, which can play a role in their manipulation of others.

✓Conduct disorder involves physical aggression and violating the basic rights of others.

Tourette's disorder

More common in males with >1 year of symptoms and occurs before 18 years of age.

Hx/PE: Multiple <u>motor</u> tics (blinking and head shaking), and <u>vocal</u> tics (including coughing, cussing, and throat clearing). Can be associated with OCD and ADHD.

Treatment:

- Movement disorders: **tetrabenazine**.
- For tics: risperidone or fluphenazine (dopamine antagonists).
- Depression: SSRIs.

Separation anxiety disorder

Child exhibits excessive distress when parental figure is not present. Usually occurs between 7 months and 3 years of age. Is normal behavior until age three and considered part of normal development. A firm diagnosis cannot be confirmed until after the age of three.

Diagnosis: Clinical diagnosis.

Treatment:

- Child counseling and behavioral therapy.
- Studies show mixed results with pharmaceutical therapy.

Bereavement in children

Can present differently depending on the child's age. It is normal that siblings will have different responses to death.

Treatment: Encourage a child to express his emotions and sadness. It is important to allow a child to completely mourn the deceased.

Selective mutism

Mutism in certain situations such as in front of teachers, certain situations, or unfamiliar people.

Personality disorders

*Personality disorders are a class of mental disorders that present as maladaptive behavior patterns. These disorders present early in life and are inflexible.

Cluster A personality disorders: "the weird"

➤ **Paranoid**
Suspicious, mistrustful, isolated, and secretive. Patients are usually emotionally odd and might have legal action against other people.

➤ **Schizoid**
Isolation, solitary, lack of close friends, emotionally distant, and no desire for close friendships.

➤ **Schizotypal**
Magical thinking, odd and eccentric behavior, and increased social anxiety. Behavior is not severe enough to be classified as schizophrenia.

Cluster B personality disorders: "the wild"

➤ **Histrionic**
Needs to be the center of attention, emotional, attention seeking, and inappropriate sexualization of non-sexual relationships. Discomfort if not center of attention.

Note: histrionic personality have increased risk of developing **hypochondriac behavior.**

➤ **Narcissistic**
Grandiose sense of self, need of admiration from others, sense of entitlement, lack of empathy, and envious of others.

Note: narcissistic typically have a sense of boredom in social interactions because they are so focused on their own issues.

➤ **Antisocial**
Failure to conform to social rules, aggressive towards others, irresponsible, and must be over 18 years of age. If less than 18 years old, patient is diagnosed as having **conduct disorder**.

➤ **Borderline**
Unstable relationships, chronic feeling of emptiness, inappropriate anger, impulsive, and brief psychotic episodes.

Treatment: Lithium and psychotherapy (**dialectical behavior therapy** is <u>most</u> effective). Dialectical behavior therapy involves building of social skills and behaviors.

Note: elevated levels of lithium (>2.5 mEq/L) with AMS or seizures requires dialysis.

Cluster C personality disorders: "**the worried**"

➤ **Avoidant**
Unwilling to become involved with others, feelings of inadequacy, and shy.

➤ **Dependent**
Difficulty making daily decisions, difficulty assuming responsibility, clingy, and seeks relationships with others.

➤ **Obsessive-compulsive personality disorder (OCPD)**
Has an obsession component, preoccupied with details, rigid, orderly, and perfectionistic. Differs from **obsessive-compulsive disorder**.

Overall treatment for personality disorders:

- Individual psychotherapy (<u>best choice</u>).
- Not usually treated with chemical treatments (medications).
- β-blockers (e.g., propranolol) can help with anxiety and improve social interactions.

Note: propranolol is commonly used to treat social anxiety, essential tremors, and esophageal varices.

Defense mechanisms

➤ **Splitting**

Defense mechanism where external objects are <u>divided</u> as "all good" or "all bad." Can develop into bipolar disorder.

➤ **Regression**

Defense mechanism where patient returns to <u>earlier</u> stages of development when dealing with conflicts.

➤ **Acting out**

Defense mechanism where a person expresses an unconscious wish through <u>actions</u> to avoid consciousness of the strong negative accompanying affect.

➤ **Passive aggressive**

Defense mechanism where aggression toward others is <u>indirectly</u> expressed and usually includes stubbornness, passivity, and forgetfulness.

➤ **Sublimation**

Defense mechanism where an unacceptable impulse is <u>transformed</u> into an acceptable one.

Mood disorders

Major depression

Mood disorder present for at *least 2 weeks*, with a change in previous level of functioning.

<u>Risks</u>: elderly patients with multiple comorbidities have a greater risk of depression. Common secondary causes are hypothyroidism, dementia, and Parkinson's disease.

Hx/PE: Anhedonia, weight change, sleep change, poor concentration, feeling of worthlessness, and possible thoughts of suicidal ideations.

Diagnosis:

- Primarily a clinical diagnosis.
- May want to rule out organic causes before treatment is initiated (especially among elderly patients). Common laboratory tests include CBC, electrolytes, TSH, FT4, glucose, B12, and VDRL.
- Toxicology screening to determine if there is substance abuse.

Note: keep in mind that depression carries increased risk for development of CAD and MIs.

Treatment:

- *First step* is psychotherapy and cognitive-behavior therapy.
- *Second step* is treatment with SSRIs (*first-line medication*).
- *Third step* (if above options are not effective) is electroconvulsive therapy (ECT).
    - ECT can also be used for faster response in suicidal patients.
- If suicidal, initiate suicidal precautions and admit to psychiatric ward.
- If suicidal ideations are passive can usually manage outpatient.

Fun facts:

- ✓ Continue medication for at least 6 months after mood is stabilized.
- ✓ To avoid sexual blunting effects or weight gain, can consider bupropion.
- ✓ Bupropion also used for smoking cessation.
- ✓ Highest risk of suicide is 2 weeks after starting anti-depressants (increased energy but remain depressed).
- ✓ If suicidal, remove all weapons from household.
- ✓ Psychiatric consultation is necessary for homicidal or suicidal ideation.
- ✓ If suicidal and patient is intoxicated, need reassessment when sober.
- ✓ Never discharge an intoxicated patient.

Bipolar

Mood disorder involving experience of manic symptoms, depression, or mixed symptoms for at *least 1 week*. Can be associated with other disorders such as eating disorders, anxiety, and drug use as well as suicide (5%).

Diagnosis: Need to rule out substance abuse (urine immunoassay drug screening); especially cocaine and amphetamine.

Treatment:

- For an *acute* manic episode, can consider haloperidol (short-term treatment).
- *First line* and *long-term* treatment is lithium (decreases suicidal ideations).
    - If no relapse in 1 year, can discontinue lithium.
    - If >3 episodes, then lifelong treatment with lithium.
- *Second line long-term* therapy is valproic acid (especially if evidence of renal failure).
- If *severe* multiple episodes occur (psychotic or aggression) and not responsive to monotherapy, use combination therapy (mood stabilizer <u>plus</u> antipsychotic).
- During first trimester of pregnancy, discontinue lithium, and start haloperidol (if severe) and if not effective consider other antipsychotics or ECT.
- Lamotrigine can be used in second and third trimesters of pregnancy.
- Valproic acid (mood stabilizer) is also teratogenic.
- If depressed, can administer anti-depressants but <u>only</u> for a short-term period (2 weeks) because this can cause rapid cycling bipolar.

Note:

✓ Lithium causes nephrogenic rather than central DI.

✓ If lithium is subtherapeutic → then increase lithium dosage.

✓ If lithium is supratherapeutic → then decrease lithium dosage.

- ✓ Lithium can decrease suicide risk.
- ✓ Most common causes of **rapid cycling bipolar** are anti-depressants and hypothyroidism.

Dysthymia

Milder chronic depression that lasts most of the day and has been present for at *least 2 years*. Associated with changes in appetite, sleep, concentration, fatigue, and feelings of hopelessness.

Diagnosis:

- Clinical diagnosis (at least 2 years of <u>mild</u> levels of depressed mood).
- Need to rule out organic causes including CBC, electrolytes, glucose, B12, and TSH.

Treatment: *First line treatment* is psychotherapy followed by administration of antidepressants (SSRIs).

Note: patients do not usually require hospitalization unless they are suicidal.

Cyclothymia

Hypomanic episodes and mild depression and frequent mood swings. Symptoms must be present for at *least 2 years*.

Diagnosis: Clinical diagnosis (at least 2 years of <u>mild</u> levels of elevated mood and mild depression).

Treatment: Psychotherapy and lithium or valproic acid.

Note: divalproex is more effective than lithium.

Atypical depression

Hx/PE: Increased sleep, increased appetite, and weight gain.

Diagnosis: Clinical diagnosis (rule out above findings).

- *First-line medication* is SSRIs.
- If substantial weight gain, use bupropion.
- When and if MAOIs are used, this would be where you might consider using this medication.

Note: SSRIs are a better choice because MAOIs have greater side effects.

Seasonal affective disorder

Depression that usually occurs when days are <u>shorter</u> and subjected to less sunlight (fall and winter).

Hx/PE: Weight gain, increased sleep, and lethargy.

Treatment: Phototherapy and bupropion (less weight gain).

Postpartum blues, **postpartum depression**, and **postpartum psychosis** are obstetrics-related disorders.

Bereavement (grief)

Normal bereavement that typically occurs after the death of a loved one and includes sadness, worry about the deceased, sleep problems, tearfulness, and poor concentration. Patient might present with delusions of the deceased person, which is common.

Note: if greater than 1 year, then called major depression and treated the same way.

Diagnosis: *Usually lasts for <6 months* but can be present for longer.

Treatment:

- Supportive psychotherapy and family/friend support is the best therapy.
- If lasts longer than 8 weeks can consider SSRIs.
- Symptoms are age-dependent in children and each child can react differently.

Age-related sleep changes

Older individuals require less sleep, take longer to fall asleep, have more daytime naps, and increased early morning awakening. They also have decreased REM stages 3 and 4 sleep.

Anxiety disorders

Panic disorder

Intense anxiety that lasts less than *30 minutes* and includes at least 4 symptoms.

Hx/PE: Diaphoresis, chills, fear of dying, shortness of breath, palpitations, dizziness, nausea, chest pain, and trembling.

Diagnosis:

- Clinical diagnosis.
- When a panic disorder occurs for the first time, need to rule out; TSH, glucose levels, urinalysis, EKG, LFTs, urine toxicology, and blood alcohol levels.

Treatment:

- Cognitive behavior therapy, but not sufficient without medications.
- Can be treated with combination therapy including SSRIs (long-term) and benzodiazepines (for acute symptoms, such as alprazolam, which has a short half-life).

Note: alprazolam is also known as Xanax.

Phobias

Fear of an object or situation; resulting in avoidance.

- ➤ Specific phobia: fear of an objects, animals, heights, or vehicles.
- ➤ Social phobia: fear of public restrooms, eating in public, public speaking, specific situations, and embarrassment.

Diagnosis: Clinical history.

Treatment:

- Behavioral modification such as **desensitization exposure** and relaxation techniques.
- Medications can include SSRIs (fluoxetine).
- If *short-term* treatment is required (such as if the patient is getting on a plane the next day), then lorazepam is a better option.

Note: propranolol can be used for social phobias.

Adjustment disorder

Not a true anxiety disorder. Involves maladaptive reaction to an identifiable stressor such as school, migration, divorce, or new job.

Hx/PE: Usually occurs *within 3 months* of the stressor and remits within 6 months. Presents with anxiety, depression, or agitation.

Treatment:

- Psychotherapy and family support is the treatment of choice.
- Not usually treated with medication.

Obsessive-compulsive disorder (OCD)

Equally common in males and females. Can experience only obsession or a combination of obsession and compulsion that typically affects the patient's level of functioning. Can be associated with drug abuse and depression, but not usually associated with high suicide risk. Can also coexist with **Tourette's disorder**.

- ➤ Obsessions: thoughts that are intrusive, do not make sense, and cause the patient anxiety.
- ➤ Compulsions: rituals, checking, counting, hand-washing, and routine behaviors.

Note: obsession are the thoughts and compulsion are the actions.

Diagnosis: Clinical history.

Treatment:

- *First line non-pharmacological intervention*: cognitive behavioral psychotherapy (exposure and response prevention; which involves repetitive exposure).
- *First line medication*: SSRIs.

Post-traumatic stress disorder (PTSD)

Usually occurs after a traumatic event such as war or a tragic death and lasts >1 month.

- **Acute stress disorder**: lasts *more than 2 days* but l*ess than one month*.
- **PTSD**: symptoms last *more than 1 month*.

Hx/PE: Individuals have been exposed to a stressor that causes fear or helplessness. May re-experience the event and avoid things such as; people, situations, or objects that remind them of the event. Affects daily functioning level.

Diagnosis: Clinical diagnosis. Need to rule out depression and substance abuse.

Treatment:

- *Acute* symptoms: benzodiazepines.
- *Long-term*: combination of SSRIs (*first-line therapy*), group counseling, and relaxation techniques.
- Long-term psychodynamic psychotherapy has not been shown to be an effective stand-alone treatment.

Generalized anxiety disorder (GAD)

Excessive worrying about life events that lasts *at least 6 months*. Not related to any single event.

Hx/PE: Tachypnea, tachycardia, anxiety, and sweating.

Treatment:

- *First line* includes cognitive behavior therapy, psychotherapy, and relaxation therapy.

- SSRIs (*first-line medication*) and buspirone (*second-line medication*) or venlafaxine.

Somatoform disorders

Somatization disorder

Physical symptoms with no medical explanation for at *least 6 months*. More common in young women and usually has a psychological component. Patients with this disorder are concerned about medical health.

Diagnosis:

- A controversial diagnosis that includes 4 pain symptoms, 1 pseudoneurologic symptom, 1 sexual dysfunction, and 2 gastrointestinal symptoms. Symptoms do not have to all be present at same time.
- Physical complaints with negative diagnostic work-up.
- Ruling out organic causes, which often times can be complicated.

Treatment: *Best treatment* is cognitive behavior therapy, which is difficult to treat.

Hypochondriac

Patients feel they have a specific disease/s despite constant reassurance and intensive laboratory work-ups. Can be associated with **histrionic personality disorder**.

Diagnosis:

- Need to rule out secondary stressors.
- Need to rule out pathology to conclude hypochondriasis.

Treatment: Frequent office visits (brief monthly visits), single primary doctor, and reassurance.

Conversion

Affects a wide variety of <u>motor</u> or <u>sensory</u> functions, including paralysis, gait disturbance, weakness, disturbances of consciousness, visual loss, or pseudoseizures. Symptoms are <u>not</u> caused by any medical or psychiatric condition. Symptoms may resolve over time.

Hx/PE: Associated with **La Belle indifference**, where the patient is <u>not</u> concerned about the impairment.

Diagnosis: Clinical diagnosis, after ruling out our pathology, such as, electrolyte imbalances, strokes, brain tumors, and head hemorrhages.

Treatment: Psychotherapy, physical therapy, and hypnosis.

Body dysmorphic disorder

Preoccupation with body image including excessive obsession with physical appearance. Can include any body part ranging from breasts, body weight, nose, hair, and nails.

Diagnosis:

- Clinical diagnosis (enquiring about frequent mirror watching is helpful in diagnostic questioning).
- Can be associated with OCD and social anxiety disorder.

Treatment:

- Refer to a physiatrist for cognitive behavioral therapy, especially if there is profound distress.
- High dose SSRIs can be effective, but only for some patients.

Factitious disorder

Faking illness, intentional or deliberately producing symptoms, demanding treatment, and playing a sick role for attention. Can be either physiological symptoms or psychological symptoms. Commonly used substances are insulin and thyroxine.

Hx/PE: Often history of employment in healthcare, with an ultimate goal of gaining hospital admission. Patients are very concerned with treatment plan (unlike malingering).

Diagnosis:

- Must always exclude organic causes.
- For example, if the condition is hypoglycemia, measure insulin (high), pro-insulin (low), and C-peptide levels (low).

Treatment:

- No specific treatment other than psychotherapy.
- SSRIs might help manage underlying problems.

Note:

✓ Factitious disorder was formerly known as **Münchausen syndrome**.

✓ **Münchausen by proxy**: if symptoms are induced into a secondary party, such as a baby.

Malingering

Conscious production of signs and symptoms for obvious secondary gains. Could be used for obtaining gains at work, school, criminal activity, or personal financial gains. Malingering is <u>not</u> a mental illness.

Diagnosis:

- Discrepancy between patient's complaints and physical examination and/or laboratory results.
- Look for patients that are more concerned with personal gains and less concerned with treatment.

Treatment: Confront patient about the outcome.

Disruptive and conduct disorders

➤ **Kleptomania**: repeatedly stealing items to relieve anxiety. Often known to return items at a later time.

➤ **Pyromania**: repeatedly lighting fires with no evidence of personal gain.

➤ **Pathologic gambling:** obsession with gambling, despite loss or negative consequences.

Human sexuality

➤ **Sexual identity**
Genetically male or female, biological characteristics, and external genitalia.

➤ **Sexual orientation**
Sexual impulses: heterosexuality, homosexuality, asexuality, or bisexuality.

➤ **Gender role**
Inner sense of gender identity.

➤ **Gender identity**
Maleness or femaleness.

➤ **Sexual aversion disorder**
Avoidance of all or almost all, genital sexual contact with sexual partner.

➤ **Masturbation**
Normal behavior. The majority of men and women masturbate.

Treatment: Only problematic when it interferes with daily functioning. SSRIs medication can decreases sexual drive.

➤ **Homosexuality**
Not considered a mental illness unless patient becomes unhappy with his or her orientation.

Sexual dysfunctions

Impotence

Inability to attain or maintain an erection during the course of sexual activity.

Diagnosis:

- *First step* is to determine organic or psychological impotence.
- *Best questions* to ask are if they have morning erections and their ability to masturbate.
- Order: CBC, electrolytes, TSH, fasting glucose, lipid profile, testosterone, ABI, pelvic Doppler, and pelvic examination.

Treatment:

- Physiological impotence: psychotherapy.
- Organic impotence: treat underlying problem.

Premature ejaculation

Ejaculation before or shortly after penetration.

Treatment: Psychotherapy, behavioral therapy, and SSRIs.

Vaginismus

Vaginismus is a sexual pain disorder that consists of involuntary muscle contraction of outer vagina. Common in women with sexual abuse, trauma, and rigid religious upbringing.

Diagnosis: Rule out primary causes with hCG, STDs, urinalysis, pelvic exam, and pelvic ultrasound.

Treatment: Kegel exercises, lubricants, and dilator therapy.

Dyspareunia

Pain during sexual intercourse due to psychological or medical causes.

Diagnosis:

- Rule out primary causes (PID, endometriosis, uterine cysts, vaginitis, or STDs).
- Order: pelvic exam, Pap smear, STD panel, urinalysis, and pelvic ultrasound.

Treatment: Psychotherapy, dilator therapy, and lubricants.

Paraphilia types

*Diagnosis of paraphilia: Occurs for *more than 6 months* and causes impairment of functioning.

*Treatment of all paraphilia: If severe, can administer psychotherapy and SSRIs (decreases sexual drive) or anti-androgens.

➤ **Sadism**
Likes to <u>induce</u> psychological or physical pain and suffering to a victim.

➤ **Masochism**
Behavior involving <u>receiving</u> pain, humiliation, and physical or mental abuse.

➤ **Pedophilia**
Sexual arousal or urges directed at <u>prep</u>ubescent children.

➤ **Frotteurism**
Rubbing of pelvis or erect penis against a non-consenting person.

➤ **Transvestic fetishism**
Cross-dressing for sexual gratification. Usually found in heterosexual males.

➤ **Exhibitionism**
Exposure of genitals to strangers.

➤ **Fetishism**
Achieves sexual pleasure from non-living objects.

Sleep disorders

Narcolepsy

Sleeping multiple times a day (at least 3 times per weeks for 3 months). Excessive daytime sleepiness, frequently occurring in young adults (early 20s).

Diagnosis: Clinical diagnosis or **polysomnography** (sleep study).

Treatment:

- *First-line treatment* (non-medication) is forced naps during the day and avoid alcohol or illicit drug use.
- **Modafinil** (*first-line medication*) helps maintain alertness and low abuse potential.

Insomnia

Inability to initiate or maintain sleep, common in anxiety disorders, panic disorder, depression, and bereavement. More common in women.

Diagnosis: Rule out depression.

Treatment:

- *First step*: relaxation techniques and behavioral therapy (sleep hygiene techniques such as going to bed and waking up at the same time, avoiding alcohol, caffeinated beverages, and avoid daytime naps).
- Sleeping medications if above techniques are ineffective.
- Elderly patients consider non-pharmacological treatment such as relaxation techniques and behavioral therapy.

Sleep attacks

Irresistible sleepiness and feels refreshed upon awakening.

Cataplexy

Sudden loss of muscle tone. Considered pathognomonic and precipitated by loud noises and emotions.

Hypnogogic

Hallucinations while going to sleep.

Hypnopompic

Hallucinations when awakening.

Sleep paralysis

Patient is awake but unable to move.

Psychotic disorders

Brief psychotic disorder

Usually occurs after a stressful event and episodes can last *from 1 day to 1 month*.

Hx/PE: Requires one or more of the following characteristics: delusions, hallucinations, disorganized speech, or catatonic behavior.

Diagnosis:

- *First step* prior to diagnosis is ruling out all substance abuse (urine immunoassay is preferred test) and blood alcohol levels.
- Also necessary to rule out CBC, electrolytes, serum ammonium, glucose levels, UA, TSH, VDRL, HIV, and epilepsy.

Treatment: Psychotherapy and antipsychotic medications.

Note: common recreational drugs that can cause psychotic symptoms are cocaine, PCP, and LSD.

Schizophreniform

Symptoms last for *more than 1 month but less than 6 months.*

Hx/PE: Delusions, hallucinations, disorganized speed, poor grooming, social withdrawal, and grossly disorganized behavior.

Diagnosis: The same work-up as specified for schizophrenia. What distinguishes the two disorders is the timeframe.

Treatment: Psychotherapy and antipsychotic medications.

Note: negative symptoms are associated with muscarinic receptors, and positive symptoms are associated with dopamine receptors.

Schizophrenia

Symptoms *last >6 month*s. Worst prognosis is associated with early diagnosis, family history, and negative symptoms.

Hx/PE: Delusions, hallucinations, disorganized speech, poor grooming, social withdrawal, and grossly disorganized behavior. Not usually related to mood disorders such as depression.

Types:

➤ **Paranoid schizophrenia**: most common type of schizophrenia, characterized by delusions or hallucination and later onset (best prognosis).

➤ **Catatonic schizophrenia:** characterized by psychomotor disturbances including rigidity, stupor, and mutism.

➤ **Disorganized schizophrenia**: early age of onset and characterized by disinhibited behaviors, "appearing disheveled," and bizarre emotional responses.

➤ **Residual schizophrenia**: lack of positive symptoms (hallucinations and delusions) and increased negative symptoms such as flat affect, poor grooming, and social withdrawal (poor prognosis).

➤ **Undifferentiated schizophrenia**: does not meet the criteria for other types of schizophrenia.

Diagnosis:

- Always order urine toxicology and blood alcohol levels.
- Order: CBC, electrolytes, ammonia levels, TSH, HIV, VDRL, and glucose levels.
- Head MRI: increased ventricular space and decrease in brain mass.

Note:

✓ Negative symptoms (worse prognosis).

✓ Treatment of persistent negative symptoms with **social skills training**.

Treatment:

- If acutely psychotic or at risk of harming self or others, first step is to hospitalize and consider use of benzodiazepines and IM haloperidol.
- *Long-term* treatment, begin with atypical antipsychotics (fewer side effects).
- Clozapine is used when patients do not respond to adequate trials of typical or atypical medications. However, never use as first-line treatment because of side effects (requires regular CBC monitoring for agranulocytosis).
- If clozapine fails, then ECT is indicated.
- If develops Parkinson's-like syndrome, the next best step is to decrease dose or change medications. If not helpful, then consider benztropine.
- Haloperidol decanoate and fluphenazine decanoate are intramuscular and only require administration a few times a month. Long-acting depot medication can be helpful in managing antipsychotic medications, if patient is non-compliant or forgets to take medications.

- Antipsychotics can cause metabolic syndrome (increased weight, lipids, and glucose levels).

Note: homicidal or suicidal patients can be hospitalized against their will.

Schizoaffective

<u>Both</u> psychotic and mood symptoms (e.g., depression). The mood disorder is what differentiates this disorder from schizophrenia.

Diagnosis: Diagnosis of exclusion: CBC, electrolytes, TSH, glucose, HIV, ammonia levels, and head MRI.

Treatment: Psychotherapy, cognitive behavior therapy, and antipsychotics.

Delusional disorder

Non-bizarre or bizarre beliefs *lasting at least 1 month*. Functioning is usually not impaired in other areas of life. Hallucinations are <u>not</u> present.

Hx/PE: Delusions can be bizarre or non-bizarre in content.

Diagnosis: For diagnosis to be made delusions cannot have prominent hallucinations.

Treatment: Psychotherapy and atypical antipsychotics are first-line therapies.

Trichotillomania

Impulse-control disorder. Encompasses the compulsive urge to pull out one's own hair. More common in females. Most frequently associated with obsessive-compulsive, borderline, and depressive disorders.

Diagnosis: Physical examination of hair, which appears cut at different stages (if uncertain, can obtain scrape biopsy with KOH).

Treatment:

- Treatment of underlying disorder with habit reversal training, psychotherapy or behavioral therapy.

- No medications specifically have been approved for trichotillomania (maybe TCAs or SSRIs).

Dissociative fugue

Sudden identity disturbance that is usually precipitated after traveling away from home. Patient presents with inability to recall own past.

Dissociative identity disorder

Also known as **personality disorder**. Identity disturbance with the presence of two or more distinct identities or personality states.

Dissociative amnesia

Commonly caused by a stressful event that precipitates amnesia and memory loss.

Pseudodementia

Most commonly caused secondary to depression.

Diagnosis: Order the following tests: CBC, electrolytes, vitamin B12, TSH, glucose levels, and VDRL (rule out possible causes with labs and imaging tests).

Treatment: Psychotherapy and SSRIs.

Eating disorders

Anorexia

More frequent in teenage girls and individuals of higher social class. Failure to maintain normal body weight and preoccupied with gaining weight. Diet restrictions, excessive exercise, and underweight.

Arrhythmia is *most common* cause of death.

Hx/PE: History of fasting, laxatives, and diuretic abuse. Patients commonly deny their condition and are concerned with appearance and frequently examine themselves. Classically can present with osteoporosis, amenorrhea, hair loss, and purging.

Diagnosis:

- Clinical diagnosis: low BMI (<18.5), hypotension, bradycardia, "lanugo hair," and edema.
- *First*, order EKG and serial electrolytes (*most dangerous complications*).
- Rule out depression, which is a common association.

Treatment:

- *First step*: correct electrolyte abnormalities, if necessary.
- Start high calorie diet and monitor electrolyte abnormalities (serial electrolytes), as hypophosphatemia is the most dangerous complication.
- *First-line and long-term treatment*: SSRIs (fluoxetine), psychotherapy, multiple discipline approach, and behavioral therapy.

Note: SSRIs have some weight gaining properties.

Indications for hospitalizing patients with anorexia:

- ➤ Severe electrolyte abnormalities.
- ➤ Rhythm disturbance.
- ➤ Suicidal ideation.
- ➤ Bradycardia.

➤ Altered mental status.

➤ BMI < 18.5.

Note:

✓ Bupropion is contraindicated because it lowers seizure threshold and further decreases weight.

✓ The electrolyte imbalance is what can lead to seizures, AMS, and arrhythmias.

Bulimia nervosa

Frequent binge eating, purging, overeating, misuse of laxatives and diuretics, and excessive exercise.

Hx/PE: Occurs later in adolescence than anorexia nervosa, often present with normal weight, and previous history of obesity. Look for enlarged parotid gland and enamel erosion (secondary to induced vomiting).

Diagnosis:

- Order: CBC (rule out anemia), electrolytes (possible: low potassium, chloride, and sodium), ABG (possible metabolic alkalosis), and EKG (possible arrhythmias).

- Can have elevated amylase and metabolic alkalosis from chronic vomiting.

  - If vomiting, possibility of metabolic alkalosis.

  - If enemas or laxatives, possibility of metabolic acidosis.

Treatment:

- *First step* is to correct electrolyte and metabolic abnormalities.

- SSRIs and psychotherapy.

Note: bulimic patients usually do not require hospitalization unless severe electrolytes abnormalities.

Psychogenic polydipsia

Excessive intake of water that is secondary to psychiatric disorder.

Hx/PE: Polyuria, vomiting, diarrhea, difficulty concentrating, electrolyte abnormalities, and confusion.

Diagnosis:

- Need to rule out antipsychotic medication (lithium), which can induce diabetes insipidus.
- Measure electrolytes (sodium levels), urine osmolality, urine sodium, and serum osmolality.
- **Water deprivation test** (normalization of both urine and serum osmolality).

Treatment: Decrease water intake and psychotherapy.

Antipsychotic medication side effects

Acute dystonia (hours–days)

Hx/PE: Muscle spasms, laryngeal spasms, and torticollis.

Treatment:

- First step is to reduce medication.
- IM administration of 2 mg of fast-active **benztropine** (anticholinergic and partial dopamine agonist).
  - If severe, would administer IM benztropine rather than oral benztropine.
- IM anti-histamines (diphenhydramine) or trihexyphenidyl.

Note: levodopa is less effective than benztropine.

Akathisia (weeks)

Hx/PE: Generalized restlessness, rocking, and inability to relax.

Treatment: Reduce dose, use beta blockers, and switch to atypical (newer) medications.

Tardive dyskinesia (rare before 6 months).

Hx/PE: Abnormal involuntary head, limb, and trunk movements. Oral/facial movements are very common.

Treatment: Switch to atypical antipsychotics (clozapine has the lowest risk).

Neuroleptic malignant syndrome (NMS)

Caused by anti-psychotic medication toxicity (decreased dopamine). Can also happen after stopping treatment with levodopa.

Hx/PE: Fever, muscular rigidity, autonomic changes, agitation, and cognitive changes.

Diagnosis: Increased CPK levels, urinalysis (acute renal failure), and leukocytosis (are helpful in the diagnosis).

Treatment:

- ICU admission. Treatment is controversial, but there is agreement to stop the medication causing the problem.
- Consider initiating **dantrolene** (calcium blocker) or bromocriptine (partial dopamine agonist) can also be useful.
- Keep patient hydrated to avoid acute renal failure.
- If fever, cooling blankets are helpful.

Anti-psychotic medications

*Atypical anti-psychotics: risperidone, quetiapine, clozapine, and olanzapine.

Haloperidol

Mechanism: high potency antipsychotic, dopaminergic antagonism (D2 receptor), powerful antiemetic effects, and long half-life.

Usage: acute anti-psychotic, Rett syndrome, Tourette's disorder, and used for sedation.

Risk factors: avoid exposure to cold temperature when using antipsychotics.

Contraindications: do not use haloperidol in PCP patients (can exacerbate symptoms). Be careful when used in elderly patients.

Risperidone

Usage: atypical antipsychotic used to treat schizophrenia, schizophreniform, and mixed and manic states of bipolar.

Side effects:

- Weight gain, diabetes, tardive dyskinesia, and NMS.
- Hyperprolactinemia secondary to dopamine antagonism pathway.
  - Includes amenorrhea, galactorrhea, sexual dysfunction, irregular menstrual periods, and infertility.

Clozapine

➤ Use clozapine when other antipsychotics fail.

➤ If clozapine fails than attempt ECT.

➤ Patients who develop fever or cold-like systems will need to stop medication, since medication carries a high risk of agranulocytosis.

➤ Patient will need weekly CBC monitoring.

Side effects: high risk of agranulocytosis, weight gain, diabetes, and hypercholesterolemia.

Note:

✓ Clozapine has minimal involvement in movement disorders.

✓ If a medication causes weight gain, it's also likely to cause DM and hyperlipidemia.

Olanzapine

Side effects: increased incidence of diabetes, hyperlipidemia, and weight gain.

Ziprasidone

Side effects: mild sedation but does <u>not</u> cause significant weight gain. However, causes GI symptoms and prolonged QT-interval (also seen in calcium depletion).

Note: patients with history of arrhythmia such avoid ziprasidone.

Quetiapine

Side effects: associated with less weight gain and has fewer extrapyramidal side effects than other antipsychotics.

Dantrolene

A calcium blocker used to treat NMS and malignant hyperthermia.

Benztropine

Mechanism: anticholinergic and partial dopamine agonist.

Usage: Parkinson's disease and acute extrapyramidal symptoms (helps with muscle rigidity and tremors).

Side effects: benztropine is contraindicated if patient has acute-angle glaucoma.

Valproate

➤ Mood stabilizer used for mania, mixed states, and rapid-cycling bipolar disorder.

➤ Commonly used when lithium is contraindicated (renal failure and thyroid pathology).

Side effects: hepatotoxicity, weight gain, and extremely contraindicated during pregnancy because inhibits folic acid.

Lithium toxicity

Side effects: tremors, nephrotoxic DI, teratogenic, and thyroid function abnormalities.

Diagnosis: Check therapeutic levels; however, side effects can also occur at therapeutic levels.

Treatment: The best approach is to decrease dosage.

Note:

- ✓ Has drug interactions with many medications including NSAID's, thiazides, and ACEIs.
- ✓ If lithium levels of ≥4 mEq/L or ≥2.5 mEq/L with severe neurological symptoms, this is an indication for dialysis

Lamotrigine

Usage: can use to treat bipolar disorder in pregnant women in second and third trimesters. Use ECT in first trimester.

Side effects: Stevens-Johnson syndrome (SJS).

Antimetics

Scopolamine

Mechanism of action: anti-cholinergic agent.

Usage: used for nausea, vomiting, and prophylaxis for motion sickness.

Side effects: increases sympathetic system.

Ondansetron (Zofran)

Mechanism of action: serotonin antagonist.

Usage: is the most potent antiemetic drug available, and is very effective for chemotherapy-induced vomiting. Is available in both oral and IV forms.

Metoclopramide (Reglan)

Mechanism of action: anti-dopamine (D2 receptors).

Usage: as an antiemetic and helpful to increase gastric mobility. Medication is safe during pregnancy and can be used for motion sickness.

Side effects: can cause Parkinson's-like side effects and acute dystonia. If develop acute dystonia treat with IV diphenhydramine or IV benzotropine.

Prochlorperazine (Phenergan)

Mechanism of action: anti-dopamine (D2 receptors).

Usage: nausea, vertigo, and vomiting.

Side effects: extrapyramidal reactions cause neuroleptic side effects such as akathisia, which can be treated with benztropine or lorazepam.

Diphenhydramine

Mechanism of action: anti-histamine.

Usage: effective for motion sickness, pruritus, allergic reactions, opiate withdrawal, nausea, and vomiting.

Side effects: avoid in elderly patients, can cause sedation, hypertension, and altered mental status.

Note: discontinue anti-histamines when flying, driving, diving, or using machinery.

Anti-depressant medications

Selective serotonin reuptake inhibitors (SSRIs)

<u>Mechanism</u>: inhibit serotonin reuptake and are primary metabolized by the liver.

Treatment:

- *First-line medication* for depression, general anxiety, and OCD.
- Continue medication use for at least 6 months after depression has subsided.
- Patients who develop **serotonin syndrome**: use IV fluids and benzodiazepine (reduce muscle rigidity).

<u>Side effects</u>:

- ➤ Decreased libido, weight gain, and serotonin syndrome.
- ➤ Need to ask about history of hypomania or mania, as SSRIs can cause manic states.
- ➤ Patients with a previous history of manic states need to be placed on a mood stabilizer before starting SSRIs (anti-depressants).
- ➤ Undesired sexual side effects, switch to bupropion.
- ➤ If not effective or unfavorable side effects after 8 weeks, switch to a different antidepressant within the same family.
- ➤ SSRIs are safe in **pregnancy**, except for paroxetine.

Note: need a washout period of 5 weeks when switching from phenelzine (MAOI) to SSRIs to avoid serotonin syndrome (can happen with conversion from MOA-B to SSRIs or TCAs).

Fluoxetine

Associated with sexual side effects including decreased libido and delayed orgasm. If develop side effects such as weight gain, continue medication with re-evaluation in 4 weeks, as side effects often improve over time.

Fluvoxamine

An SSRI commonly used to treat OCD.

<u>Side effects</u>: can cause antiplatelet effects and should be discontinued 1 week prior to surgery.

MAOIs

<u>Usage</u>: can be used to treat atypical depression.

<u>Side effects</u>: **hypertension crisis** can occur with ingestion of tyramine, aged cheeses, over-the-counter cold medications (anti-histamines), and red wine. **Serotonin syndrome** can also occur when SSRIs are combined.

<u>If overdose:</u> treat with IV labetalol.

Tricyclic antidepressants (TCAs)

<u>Mechanism</u>: inhibits NE and serotonin re-uptake.

<u>Usage</u>: *imipramine*: enuresis or *amitriptyline*: chronic pain.

<u>Side effects</u>: can cause mydriasis, coma, seizures, constipation, confusion, orthostatic hypotension, dry mouth, flushing, and blurry vision.

Diagnosis for overdose:

- Need to monitor for arrhythmias (EKG) and seizures.
- Need baseline EKG prior to treatment.
    - EKG: test for prolonged widen QRS complex, prolonged PR, and QT-interval.
- Foley catheter will usually show large volumes of urine (polyuria).

Treatment for overdose:

- *First step* is sodium bicarbonate (alkalinize urine and prevention of arrhythmias) and benzodiazepines (seizures prophylaxis and treatment).

- If overdose leads to ventricular arrhythmias, lidocaine is the drug of choice.

Bupropion

An atypical anti-depressant that can aid in smoking cessation (need to gradually discontinue smoking during the second week of treatment).

Side effects: weight loss and contraindicated for use by patients with seizures (lowers seizure threshold).

Note: bupropion is not recommended for anorexic patients.

Buspirone

➤ A second-line therapy for GAD (excessive worrying about real-life circumstances).

➤ *First-line medications* for treatment of generalized anxiety are SSRIs.

Trazodone

Also a strong sedative and commonly used for severe insomnia associated with depression.

Side effects: increased priapism. If lasts longer than 2-3 hours, first attempt use of ice packs then consider phenylephrine or epinephrine injections.

Note: erection lasting longer than 3 hours is a **medical emergency**.

Mirtazapine (Remeron)

Usage: for depressed patients who require weight gain.

Side effects: weight gain, which makes this a good alternative medication for facilitating weight gain in cancer patients.

Venlafaxine (Effexor)

Mechanism: atypical antidepressant that inhibits SSRI uptake and NE reuptake.

Usage: depression, anxiety, phobias, OCP, and panic disorders.

Side effects: elevated blood pressure.

Electroconvulsive therapy (ECT)

➤ Good option for depression not resolved by standard treatments.

➤ An option for bipolar in **pregnant** patients, as lithium and valproic acid are contraindicated.

➤ Good for bipolar patients who are breast-feeding.

➤ Good for suicidal patients.

Side effects: headaches and "transient memory loss".

Benzodiazepines

Benzodiazepines

Mechanism of action: GABA receptors (increase frequency of chloride ions).

➤ Used for insomnia, acute anxiety, night terrors, delirium tremors, and sleepwalking.

➤ Supportive treatment for alcohol withdrawal, cocaine overdose, and amphetamine overdose.

Side effects: dependency and sedation. Use of narcotics may need oxygen supplementation if hypoxia and confusion develops.

Note:

✓ Need to decrease dose in elderly patients and cannot abruptly change dosages.

✓Need to warn patients about driving and machinery as can cause drowsiness.

Lorazepam

Can be used in the management of severe anxiety, DTs, and acute agitation.

Note: lorazepam can be administered for alcohol and benzodiazepine withdrawal.

Alprazolam

Need to slowly wean patients off benzodiazepines, as these medications can be life threatening. Also known as **Xanax**.

➤ For acute anxiety, panic disorder, insomnia, and phobias (but not usually first-line treatment because of secondary effects).

➤ Can be helpful for acute episodes, but rarely used for long-term symptom control.

Midazolam

➤ Used orally or rectally for conscious sedation for minor procedures (endoscopy).

➤ Patient can still control airways.

Hormonal abnormalities

➤ Major depression

Decreased serotonin and norepinephrine.

➤ Psychosis

Increased dopamine.

➤ Found in violent or impulsive people

Decreased serotonin levels.

➤ Alzheimer's disease

Decreased acetylcholine.

➤ Parkinson's disease

Decreased dopamine.

➤ Low 5-hydroxyindoleacetic acid

Associated with lack of impulse control and found in patients with OCD and intermittent explosive behavior.

Index

Index, cont'd.

divalproex 62
Donepezil 30
dorsal column medial
    lemniscus 10
dyskinesia 82
dyspareunia 71
dysthymia 62
dystonia 81

E

eceptive aphasia 40
ECT 90
Effexor 90
Ependymoma 37
epidural hematoma 3
essential tremor 35
Ethosuximide 19
expressive aphasia 40
exudative/neovascular
    degeneration 46

F

factitious disorde 68
fetal hydantoin syndrome 18
Fluorescein angiography 47
Fluoxetine 87
Fluvoxamine 88
folate deficiency 44
fugue 78
fundus photography 48

G

GAD 66
gambling 70
glaucoma 44
glioblastoma multiforme 36
grand mal 17
Guillain-Barré syndrome 27

H

Haloperidol 82

hearing test 23
hemangioblastoma 36
histrionic personality disorder. 67
Horner's syndrome 13
Huntington's disease 33
hypnogogic 74
hypnopompic 74
hypochondriac 67

I

identity disorder 78
idiopathic intracranial
    hypertension 37
impotence 71
Infantile spasms 20
insomnia 73
ischemic stroke 7

K

kleptomania 70
Korsakoff's dementia 42

L

La Belle indifference 68
labyrinthitis 22
lacunar stroke 8
Lambert-Eaton myasthenic
    syndrome 25
Lamotrigine 85
laser peripheral iridotomy 45
laser trabeculectomy 45
laser trabeculoplasty 45
lateral corticospinal tract 10
Lhermitte sign 26
lithium 85
LMN lesions 10
locked-in-syndrome 41
Lorazepam 91
Lou Gehrig' 28
lower motor neuron lesion 10

Neurology & Psychiatry In Your Pocket

Index, cont'd.

Index, cont'd.

www.ingramcontent.com/pod-product-compliance
Lightning Source LLC
Chambersburg PA
CBHW040826180526
45159CB00001B/86